THE **BLOOD SUGAR SOLUTION**

10-DAY
DETOX
DIET
COOKBOOK

THE **BLOOD SUGAR SOLUTION**

10-DAY DETOX DIET

COOKBOOK

Lose Up to 10lb in 10 Days
and Stay Healthy for Life

Dr Mark Hyman

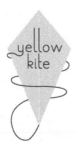

First published the USA in 2015 by Little, Brown and Company
Hachette Book Group Inc

First published in Great Britain in 2016 by Yellow Kite Books
An imprint of Hodder & Stoughton
An Hachette UK company

4

A CIP catalogue record for this title is available from the British Library.

Paperback ISBN 978 1 473 65034 3
Ebook ISBN 978 1 473 65033 6

Printed and bound in Great Britain by Clays Ltd, Elcograf S.p.A.

Hodder & Stoughton policy is to use papers that are natural, renewable and recyclable products and made from wood grown in sustainable forests. The logging and manufacturing processes are expected to conform to the environmental regulations of the country of origin.

Hodder & Stoughton Ltd
Carmelite House
50 Victoria Embankment
London EC4Y 0DZ

www.hodder.co.uk

For the generations of Americans who never learned to cook or to care for and nourish their precious human bodies, this book is for you.

Contents

THE **BLOOD SUGAR SOLUTION**

10-DAY
DETOX
DIET
COOKBOOK

What Is the 10-Day Detox Diet?

If you're one of the millions suffering from obesity, diabetes, high blood pressure, or even just plain feeling crummy as a result of the Standard American Diet (SAD), *The Blood Sugar Solution 10-Day Detox Diet* is for you. It provides a step-by-step guide for losing weight and even reversing disease. Follow it for just ten days and your life will never be the same!

The 10-Day Detox Diet outlines a way of eating that will help you reverse the food addiction brought on by the $1-trillion industrial food system—the system that turns sugar, salt, and fat into druglike foods that hook you with every bite. This steady stream of hyperprocessed, highly palatable, intensely addictive foods sabotages your brain chemistry, your waistline, and your health. The way to reclaim your health and your life starts with what I call food rehab. It means a dramatic shift, but it will provide you with the fundamental skills you need to lose weight, change your biochemistry, and kick your addiction forever!

In a recent study, Harvard professor Dr. David Ludwig explains why for the first time. It turns out that it's not overeating that makes you fat; it's being fat that makes you overeat. When you consume refined carbohydrates such as bread, rice, potatoes, pasta, and any form of sugar, you make a certain kind of fat called *visceral adipose tissue* (VAT). This is no ordinary fat. It is super fat. Hungry fat. Dangerous fat. This fat starts an inexorable cascade that leads to obesity. It's like falling down an icy slope where it's almost impossible to stop yourself. We ordinary mortals are no match for this hungry fat.

Here's what happens: VAT cells suck up much of the available fuel in your bloodstream (glucose, fats, ketones). Your body then thinks, "Oh, jeez, I am starving. I better eat more and slow my metabolism, so I don't die." The problem is that anything you eat gets sucked up into those fat cells around your belly, leading to a vicious cycle of hunger, overeating, fat storage, and a slowing down of your metabolism. No wonder we gain weight and can't lose it.

The key trigger for all of this is a hormone that we all need, albeit in moderation: insulin — the fat storage hormone.

If we make too much insulin, it drives the fuel from our blood into our fat cells. Too much insulin also does a lot of other bad things, such as cause heart attacks, high cholesterol, type 2 diabetes, cancer, and dementia.

What causes insulin to spike? Not all calories are created equal: Sugar and refined carbohydrate calories are the culprits. Most Americans eat, on average, about 152 pounds (69 kg) of sugar and 146 pounds (66 kg) of flour a year (combined, that's almost a pound (450 g) of sugar and flour per person, per day).

The Blood Sugar Solution 10-Day Detox Diet is scientifically designed to stop this vicious cycle quickly. Think of it as your ice axe and crampons to halt your descent down the slippery slope of obesity and chronic disease. It will quickly block the hormones and brain chemicals that make you hungry and crave sugar and carbs. And instead of storing fat and being burdened with a slow metabolism, you will burn fat and speed up your metabolism.

Once you enjoy all of the healing benefits of the 10-Day Detox Diet, my guess is that you'll want to incorporate many of the elements into your life. That's why I've written this cookbook: to review the principles of the program and help support you with information and recipes so you can continue on your path to good health. After all, food is medicine, and I believe you'll find that it's even more powerful than anything you will find in a pill bottle.

The recipes in this book follow the principles of the 10-Day Detox

Diet. I have also included recipes for you to enjoy when the ten days are over—during what I call the "transition phase." After all, better health doesn't start and end in ten days. It's a lifelong journey. I've set out to make that journey both doable and delicious.

PART I

THE BASICS

Many of you who have picked up this cookbook may have already read *The Blood Sugar Solution 10-Day Detox Diet* and have experienced the profound effects of resetting your metabolism using food as medicine. I hope you now are addicted not to sugar but to feeling good and you are looking for additional recipes, meal ideas, and encouragement to help you stay on track and maintain the amazing way you feel now.

1

Why Detox?

For those of you who struggle with weight, who are skinny on the outside but fat on the inside, or who have FLC (feel like crap) syndrome, food addiction is often at the root. Addiction to sugar, flour, and processed foods hijacks your life and leads to metabolic chaos—increasing cravings and hunger, slowing metabolism, and packing on belly fat. Although the idea of a detox may sound extreme, I strongly believe that it is the only way to balance your hormones and blood sugar, reduce insulin spikes, cool off inflammation, improve digestion, and boost your metabolism. Think of it as a delicious, energy-boosting, scientific method for detoxing from foods high in sugars and refined carbohydrates and processed food.

We tracked more than 600 people who tried the 10-Day Detox Diet program and found that they experienced dramatic results. On average they lost 8 pounds (3.6 kg) and 3.4 percent of their body weight, 2 inches (5 cm) off their waist, and 1 inch (2.5 cm) off their hips. Some people lost up to 10 inches (25 cm) around their waist, and up to 11 inches (27 cm) around their hips. The average drop in fasting blood sugar was 18 points. The average blood pressure fell 10 points. Even better, they had more energy, reported better sleep, and experienced improvements in their mood. They had a 62 percent reduction in symptoms from all diseases. There is no drug on the planet that can do that. One seventy-year-old man told me he lost 45 pounds (20 kg), got off 52 units of insulin, and completely reversed his diabetes. Another told me his rheumatoid arthritis went away in ten days, and yet another reported that her daily migraines had vanished. These results came not from pill bottles but from food.

In the following pages, I feature three quizzes that will help you identify if you are addicted to food in any way, or if your relationship to food is interfering with the quality of your life, or if food is doing anything other than helping you thrive and feel amazing. If so, then you need this detox. If you have *diabesity*—the continuum of metabolic damage ranging from a little belly fat to pre-diabetes to type 2 diabetes, or if you just don't feel well, then the 10-Day Detox Diet can profoundly improve your health and the quality of your life. And because I encourage you to keep track of your progress during the detox, you will see the results right away.

ARE YOU A FOOD ADDICT?

I'm fed up with the food giants and even many health professionals who perpetuate the myth that a calorie is a calorie—that the 500 calories you wolf down in a Big Mac have the same impact on your body as 500 calories of broccoli. Not all calories are equal. Calories from sugar and refined carbs spike blood sugar, trigger insulin, and lead to a cascade of hormonal and brain chemistry changes that promote fat storage, hunger, and a slow metabolism. Science also supports the notion that your Big Mac, Double Gulp, and other hyperprocessed fat, sugar, and salt bombs are addictive.

While at Yale's Rudd Center for Food Policy and Obesity, my friend and colleague Kelly Brownell, PhD, created a scientifically validated food questionnaire to help you determine whether you are a food addict. I've adapted the quiz below.

QUIZ: Are You Addicted to Food?
Ask yourself how often you experience any of these feelings and behaviors (hint: the more often you experience them, the more addicted you are):

- You consume certain foods even if you are not hungry, because of cravings.

- You worry about cutting down on certain foods.
- You feel sluggish or fatigued from overeating.
- You have spent time dealing with negative feelings from overeating certain foods, instead of spending time in important activities with family, friends, work, or recreation.
- You have had withdrawal symptoms such as agitation and anxiety when you've cut down on certain foods (do not include caffeinated drinks such as coffee, tea, or energy drinks).
- Your behavior with respect to food and eating causes you significant distress.
- Issues related to food and eating decrease your availability to function effectively (daily routine, job/school, social or family activities, health difficulties).
- You need more and more of the foods you crave to experience any pleasure or to reduce negative emotions.

If you see yourself in these clues, don't worry—you're far from alone. Millions of people in every corner of the world have fallen into the food addiction trap. The 10-Day Detox Diet helps you discover once and for all the path that leads you out of biochemical imprisonment and into food freedom. This cookbook helps support you on your journey.

DO YOU HAVE DIABESITY?

As if food addiction isn't destructive enough on its own, the industrial foods that have this druglike effect can also lead to diabesity. Type 2 diabetes now affects one in two American adults (and one in four kids).

In the following quiz, you'll discover whether you're suffering from the symptoms of pre-diabetes or type 2 diabetes—inflammation, high triglycerides, unhealthy cholesterol levels, high blood pressure, and high blood sugar. If you answer "yes" to even one of the following questions, you may already have diabesity or are headed in that direction.

QUIZ: Do I Have Diabesity?

1. Do you have a family history of diabetes, heart disease, or obesity?
2. Are you of nonwhite ancestry (African, Asian, Native American, Pacific Islander, Hispanic, Indian, Middle Eastern)?
3. Are you overweight (body mass index, or BMI, over 25)? Go to www.10daydetox.com/tools to calculate your BMI based on your weight and height.
4. Do you have extra belly fat? Is your waist circumference greater than 35 inches (88 cm) for women or greater than 40 inches (100 cm) for men?
5. Do you crave sugar and refined carbohydrates?
6. Do you have trouble losing weight on a low-fat diet?
7. Has your doctor told you that your blood sugar is a little high (greater than 100 mg/dL) or have you actually been diagnosed with insulin resistance, pre-diabetes, or type 2 diabetes?
8. Do you have high levels of triglycerides (over 100 mg/dL) or low levels of HDL ("good") cholesterol (under 50 mg/dL)?
9. Do you have heart disease?
10. Do you have high blood pressure?
11. Are you inactive (less than 30 minutes of exercise 4 times a week)?
12. Do you suffer from infertility, low sex drive, or sexual dysfunction?
13. For women: Have you had gestational diabetes or polycystic ovarian syndrome (PCOS)?

ARE YOU SICK?

You'll also want to find out just how sick you are by taking the Toxicity Quiz (adapted from the Immuno Symptom Checklist created in 1989 by Immuno Laboratories). Most of us walk around tolerating chronic symptoms (not just weight issues) that are connected to what we eat, including digestive issues, headaches, joint pain, fatigue, depression, autoimmune diseases, and more. Most of us just don't connect the dots. If we eat crap, we will feel like crap. This quiz will give you a baseline for your existing symptoms, which are indications of being toxic and inflamed. Score it now and again after you've completed the program, and you will experience for yourself, after just ten days, a dramatic difference in the way you look and feel.

For the "before" part of the questionnaire, rate each of the following symptoms based upon your health profile for the past 30 days.

Point Scale
0 = Never or almost never have the symptom
1 = Occasionally have it, effect is not severe
2 = Occasionally have, effect is severe
3 = Frequently have it, effect is not severe
4 = Frequently have it, effect is severe

Digestive Tract
_____ Nausea or vomiting
_____ Diarrhea
_____ Constipation
_____ Bloated feeling
_____ Belching or passing gas
_____ Heartburn
_____ Intestinal/stomach
   pain
Total before _____
Total after _____

Ears
_____ Itchy ears
_____ Earaches or ear infections
_____ Drainage from ear
_____ Ringing or hearing
   loss
Total before _____
Total after _____

Emotions
_____ Mood swings
_____ Anxiety, fear, or
   nervousness

_____ Anger, irritability, or
   aggressiveness
_____ Depression
Total before _____
Total after _____

Energy/Activity
_____ Fatigue or sluggishness
_____ Apathy or lethargy
_____ Hyperactivity
_____ Restlessness
Total before _____
Total after _____

Eyes
_____ Watery or itchy eyes
_____ Swollen, reddened, or
   sticky eyelids
_____ Bags or dark circles under
   eyes
_____ Blurred or tunnel vision
   (does not include near- or
   farsightedness)
Total before _____
Total after _____

Head

_____Headaches

_____Faintness

_____Dizziness

_____Insomnia

Total before _____

Total after _____

Heart

_____Irregular or skipped
heartbeat

_____Rapid or pounding
heartbeat

_____Chest pain

Total before _____

Total after _____

Joints/Muscles

_____Pain or aches in joints

_____Arthritis

_____Stiffness or limitation of
movement

_____Pain or aches in muscles

_____Feeling of weakness or
tiredness

Total before _____

Total after _____

Lungs

_____Chest congestion

_____Asthma or bronchitis

_____Shortness of breath

_____Difficulty breathing

Total before _____

Total after _____

Mind

_____Poor memory

_____Confusion or poor
comprehension

_____Poor concentration

_____Poor physical coordination

_____Indecisiveness

_____Stuttering or stammering

_____Slurred speech

_____Learning disabilities

Total before _____

Total after _____

Mouth/Throat

_____Chronic coughing

_____Gagging or frequent need
to clear throat

_____Sore throat, hoarseness, or
loss of voice

_____Swollen or discolored
tongue, gums, or lips

_____Canker sores

Total before _____

Total after _____

Nose

_____Stuffy nose

_____Sinus problems

_____Hay fever

_____Excessive mucus formation

_____Sneezing attacks

Total before _____

Total after _____

Skin

_____ Acne

_____ Hives, rashes, or dry skin

_____ Hair loss

_____ Flushing or hot flashes

_____ Excessive sweating

Total before _____

Total after _____

Weight

_____ Binge eating/drinking

_____ Craving certain foods

_____ Excessive weight

_____ Compulsive eating

_____ Water retention

_____ Underweight

Total before _____

Total after _____

Other

_____ Frequent illness

_____ Frequent or urgent urination

_____ Genital itch or discharge

Total before _____

Total after _____

Grand Total Before _____

Grand Total After _____

Key to Questionnaire

Optimal health: less than 10

Mild toxicity: 10–50

Moderate toxicity: 50–100

Severe toxicity: over 100

2

Getting Started

The antidote to your weight and health problems doesn't lie in the pharmacy—it lies, as I have always said, in the "farmacy." The foods in your farmers' market and supermarket hold the cure, and the 10-Day Detox Diet is the way to break the cycle and reset, reboot, and restore your body to good health. This companion cookbook will support you in your mission. It will help you reconnect with your kitchen and prepare real, whole, delicious meals for yourself and those you love.

There are three phases of the 10-Day Detox Diet, all keys to your lifelong success. This cookbook will enhance your experience by providing you with more than 150 mouthwatering recipes to give your metabolism a boost. Let's look at the three phases:

Phase 1, the Prep Phase: Here you'll clean out your fridge and pantry in order to set yourself up for success. Spend about two days prior to beginning your detox setting up both mentally and physically. We'll get to specific foods and ingredients in Chapter 4.

Phase 2, the 10-Day Detox: This is the actual "meat" of the program—the ten days that you'll spend resetting your biochemistry and jumpstarting the healing process.

Phase 3, the Transition Phase: Now you'll learn strategies for long-term health so you can continue to feel great after the first ten days.

I've organized the meals in this cookbook to help your body progress according to the same guidelines I outlined in *The Blood Sugar Solution 10-Day Detox Diet*. My dream is for you to follow the comprehensive program in that book and give your body the best chance to reset itself to health. However, if you've picked up this cookbook and want to start with food as your medicine, then you will still experience profound changes in your weight, health, and well-being in just ten days.

WHY 10 DAYS?

Ten days is not a magic number or a gimmicky weight-loss scheme. Most people don't realize that they are only a few days away from health and happiness. When you rapidly shift the way you eat, you can shift your hormones, brain chemistry, and biology very quickly. You can normalize your blood sugar, restore your liver and pancreas to a healthier state, and even improve your metabolism. Your body is capable of amazing things if you give it a chance. Just try it for ten days. You are capable of doing anything for that amount of time. And in exchange for a radical change in your lifestyle, I'm offering you a radical promise: that you will emerge within the first week feeling lighter, happier, more energetic, and more alive. You'll also be released from the grip of food addiction, and your body will be less toxic than it has been in years. Within this cookbook, you'll find the recipes and tools you need to free yourself from the cravings and health struggles that plague you.

WHAT TO TRACK

Throughout your ten-day journey and beyond, I encourage you to track your results. Research shows that people who track their results lose twice as much weight and do twice as well. Begin by getting a journal; it could be as simple as a notebook or a spreadsheet on your computer, whatever is convenient and works for you.

Now, what should you track? For starters, you'll want to get a baseline of all measurements. Before you begin, talk with your healthcare provider about the program if you're already on medication for high blood pressure or high blood sugar. If you are, the diet can work so quickly that your blood sugar or blood pressure may drop significantly—one patient had her sugar drop from 220 to normal in three days. So it is important to work with your doctor to adjust your medication and keep close track of these measurements. Using a home glucose monitor and blood pressure cuff can help you keep close tabs on how your body responds to this healing way of eating. Check out www.10daydetox.com/tools for my recommendations for self-tracking and monitoring devices that track weight, exercise, blood pressure, blood sugar, and more.

Here's a list of what to record, how often to recheck, and what you need to get started:

YOUR WEIGHT

Weigh yourself, without clothes, first thing in the morning after going to the bathroom. Track your weight weekly in your journal.

YOUR HEIGHT

Measure yourself in feet and inches. Write it in your journal.

YOUR WAIST SIZE

Measure the widest point around your belly button. Track this measurement weekly in your journal. You can also track your hips at the widest point around your butt.

YOUR BODY MASS INDEX (BMI)

Your BMI is your weight in kilograms divided by your height in meters squared. You can use our online calculator at www.10daydetox .com/tools or use this calculation:

BMI = weight in pounds times 703, then divided by height in inches squared

So let's use me for example: I weigh 185 pounds and am 75 inches tall. The calculation is: $185 \times 703 \div (75 \times 75)$. My BMI is 23.

This gives you a way to track whether you are normal weight, overweight, or obese. Normal BMI is less than 25, overweight is 26 to 29, and obese is over 30. However, you should take into account your waist size as well. If you weigh a lot but are a muscular bodybuilder with a small waist, you could be healthy and still have a high BMI. If you have skinny arms and legs and a skinny butt but a potbelly, you might have a normal BMI but be at risk for diabesity.

Furthermore, certain ethnic groups—such as Asians, Hispanics, Pacific Islanders, Inuits, Indians, and Middle Easterners—have diabesity at much lower BMIs. Track your BMI weekly in your journal.

YOUR BLOOD PRESSURE (optional)

Get a home blood pressure cuff and measure your blood pressure first thing every morning and write it down.

WHAT TESTS SHOULD YOU DO?

Test Your Blood Sugar Yourself

While measuring your blood sugar is optional before, during, and after the 10-Day Detox Diet, I highly recommend it. Many people think they don't have to check their blood sugar unless they are diabetic. Not so. In fact, I think it is a simple, great way for everyone to see how their body responds to what they eat.

Some of you may already have a glucose meter and know how to test your blood sugar. Others may want to get a meter at their local drugstore. The newer ones are easy to use and you can always ask your pharmacist to show you how. I like the ACCU-CHEK Aviva Blood Glucose Meter with Strips, which includes a few test strips (you may need extra).

Here is the protocol I recommend for testing:

- Measure your fasting blood sugar daily, first thing in the morning before breakfast. Ideally your fasting blood sugar should be between 70 and 80 mg/dL.
- Measure your blood sugar two hours after breakfast and two hours after dinner. Ideally your two-hour sugars should never go over 120 mg/dL. If they go over 140 mg/dL, you have pre-diabetes. If they

go over 200 mg/dL, you have type 2 diabetes. Technically this is after a 75-gram glucose load, but if they go this high on the plan you definitely have a problem. Pay attention to how they change depending on what you eat over the ten days.

Get Tested with Your Doctor

Part of what you're doing over these ten days is becoming an active partner in your health and weight loss plan, and that includes having a full understanding of your numbers and following them over time. I believe everyone should become empowered to learn about their bodies, interpret their test results, and use that information to track their progress. I strongly encourage you to consider getting basic lab tests done before and after the program. These would include the following:

- Insulin response test, which is like a two-hour glucose tolerance test, but it measures insulin as well as glucose three times: after fasting, and one and two hours after a 75-gram glucose drink.
- Hemoglobin A1c, which measures your average blood sugar over the last six weeks. Anything over 5.5 percent is considered elevated, and over 6.0 percent is diabetes.

The lab tests above can be done through your doctor and at most hospitals or laboratories, or ordered yourself through personal testing companies. For more information and detailed explanations for each of these tests, go to www.10daydetox.com/tools.

- NMR lipid (cholesterol) profile, which measures LDL, HDL, and triglycerides, as well as the particle number and, importantly, the particle size of each type of cholesterol and triglycerides. Diabesity causes you to have many small dangerous LDL and HDL cholesterol particles. This is a newer test, but I would demand it from your doctor, because the typical cholesterol tests done by most labs and doctors are out of date.

Keep a record of your initial results and then track your progress as I've outlined above. You can do this with a simple pen and paper, or you use the online tools at www.10daydetox.com/tools for tracking all your scores, measurements, and vital stats, as well as your daily experiences and feelings through the detox journal.

3

Why Cook?

With our busy lives, so many of us shy away from cooking. Between our never-ending to-do lists, demanding jobs, busy children's schedules, and perhaps less-than-stellar skills in the kitchen, cooking seems to slide down the list of priorities. But when you consider all of the benefits of making a meal, you'll be inspired to channel your inner chef. Cooking a meal for yourself, a family member, or a friend is an act of love. It's a chance to strengthen bonds, teach important life-extending skills to our children, and enrich and nourish our bodies and our souls. The food industry wants us to believe that cooking is difficult, time consuming, inconvenient, and expensive, but meals need not be complicated or time consuming to be delicious and satisfying. The science is clear. You can eat well for less money by making simple, whole, fresh food. In fact, a simple dinner for a family of four consisting of roast chicken, vegetables, and salad can cost about half of what dinner out at McDonald's would cost.

I once visited an obese sick family who had never cooked. They lived on food stamps and disability allowance. With one simple cooking lesson and a guide from the Environmental Working Group called "Good Food on a Tight Budget," they started cooking. In the first year, the mother lost over 100 pounds (45 kg), the father lost 45 pounds (20 kg), and their teenage son lost 40 pounds (18 kg). Unfortunately, the son has since gained the weight back because the only jobs for teenagers in the food desert where they live are at a fast food chain. It's like sending an alcoholic to work in a bar! These days over 50 percent of meals are consumed outside the home, but it's my goal to get you to reconnect with your kitchen and the bounty of benefits it offers.

The reasons are simple. With today's toxic food environment—the slick combination of sugar, salt, and fat that's pumped into a wide range of packaged food—our genes (and our jeans) are overwhelmed. Our taste buds have been assaulted and our tongues and brains adapt by craving even more of these toxins. However, our hormones and biochemical pathways haven't adapted to this style of eating. The result is that nearly 70 percent of Americans are overweight, and obesity rates in the United States are expected to top 42 percent by the end of the next decade (up from only 13 percent in 1960).

Today one in two Americans has either pre-diabetes or diabetes. In less than a decade the rate of pre-diabetes or diabetes in teenagers has risen from 9 percent to 23 percent. Perhaps even more shocking, 37 percent of kids at a normal weight have pre-diabetes and one or more cardiovascular risk factors such as high blood pressure, high cholesterol, or high blood sugar, because even though overly processed food doesn't necessarily make you fat, it can make you sick. In addition to raising the risk for chronic, life-threatening diseases, the sad truth is that obese children will earn less, suffer more, and die younger.

But all of this can be reversed, and the cure lies in your kitchen. It also lies in your supermarket, not just with the fresh foods in the produce aisle, but also with some of the packaged foods that are tucked away in the middle. Healthy foods such as nuts and nut butters and nondairy milks are hidden gems in the middle aisles of the store. There are even brands making healthy packaged meals using quality ingredients from real, whole food—for those nights when cooking truly is out of the question. And some companies have created high-quality, delicious, affordable, and healthy frozen meals.

By purchasing these foods, you're going to transform yourself, but you're also helping to transform the food industry one small choice at a time. The problems are global, but the solution is as local as your fork! The movement is already under way, being driven by those of us who are fed up with Big Food poisoning our taste buds and our bodies. You have the power to join the movement, and it doesn't take a picket line or even a huge pocketbook. All it takes is voting with your wallet at the grocery store.

It's time for a revolution. Cooking real food is a revolutionary act. Without kitchen skills, we have lost the means to care for ourselves. Our children will grow up without these survival tactics, and their children will face the same fate—not being able to identify common fruits and vegetables, and not realizing where food comes from. I urge you to reconsider whatever notions you have about cooking—that it costs too much, that it's too hard, that it takes too long. The recipes within this cookbook are designed to challenge these myths, to reunite you with real food, and to delight your taste buds while nourishing your body. As an added bonus, you may find, as I do, that cooking can be fun and relaxing.

THE FAMILY KITCHEN

There is a reason why today's modern kitchens are open and inviting: People love to gather in the kitchen. It's the place for nourishing your body and your relationships. It's a space in which to bond with your children while teaching them valuable life skills.

Sadly, today's overscheduled families have a difficult time slowing down and tapping into this sacred space and all the wonders it has to offer. If this sounds familiar, I encourage you to reclaim your kitchen and your family time. Look carefully at your days and examine where you spend your time. Are you watching TV at night? Spending an hour on Facebook and Instagram? Many people spend more time watching someone cook on television than actually cooking. After close consideration, you may find that you can reorganize your to-do list, revisit your viewing habits, shut off your computer, and recover your precious time.

What we need is a lifestyle that makes cooking easy, inviting, and fun. And whether you're preparing food together or passing it around the family table, dinner is a wonderful time to reconnect, get the day's download, share laughs, and discuss important events. Start your new ritual by making your kitchen as warm and inviting as possible. Create a family playlist that puts everyone in a good mood. Invest in terrific lighting. Change your curtains. Open your windows. Put stools by the counter, or pillows on your chairs. Make the kitchen a place you and your family *want* to gather.

Once you set up the environment for success, let the fun begin! If you're new to cooking or your skills have gotten rusty, don't aim for perfection with your first recipe—experiment and practice. Start with one of my more basic recipes, with only a few ingredients, and work your way up to something more complex. Enlist help from family members—drag your kids away from their video games and ask them to measure ingredients, pull food from the fridge, or even chop veggies if they're ready to take on this task. Decide on meals together to get everyone excited about what's in store.

I encourage you to start your own family traditions around cooking and enjoying meals together. One of my favorite things to do with my kids is to hang out in the kitchen, chopping vegetables, telling stories, catching up, cooking, and anticipating sharing a great meal together. Once you get in the habit of nourishing your family life in this way, you'll never want to return to solo dining out of plastic containers and take-out boxes.

DINNER CONVERSATIONS: CREATING MAGIC AT MEALTIME

Want to make a great meal even better? Share it over an inspired dinner conversation.

Life coach Lauren Zander (cofounder of the Handel Group and creator of the Handel Method) has a fantastic mealtime tradition I'd like to share. She calls it "Creating a Conversation."

It works like this: At the start of the meal, your family or dinner guests suggest a potential question to be answered by each person at the table.

Everyone must agree on the question. Once a question is decided upon, everyone at the table *must* answer. The magic happens as everyone shares about themselves and connects with one another. You will get to know your family and friends on a deeper level.

To help you get started, here's a list of some of our favorite dinner conversations:

- What's your favorite thing about the person sitting to your right? Why?
- How would you describe the person on your left to someone who had never met them before?
- What's your favorite thing about the current season (winter, spring, summer, or fall)? What makes it special to you? What's your best memory from this season?
- What's something you can confess that nobody at the table knows about you?
- If you could pick any career in the world, regardless of ability or age, what would it be? Why?
- Dream up a new career for everyone at the table—if you could pick any job in the world for them, what would it be? Why?
- What's a city, town, or country you've never seen that you'd like to visit? Why?
- What's your very first memory of life?
- Tell the story of your first true love. Who was it? How old were you? What happened? Do you know anything about where they are right now?
- If the house was on fire and you could save just one of your possessions, what would it be? Why?
- If you could change one thing about yourself, what would it be? Why?
- What's the most embarrassing thing that has ever happened to you? What did you learn from it?
- If you could give the person to your left a superpower, what would it be? Why?

- What's something you saw, heard, or experienced this week that touched you?
- Tell a story of someone you deeply loved. Let us know what made that person special.
- What do you love most about your life? Why?
- What's something you do that makes you feel powerful? Why?
- Everyone has their own magic gift (e.g., finding a parking spot, intuitively knowing when someone important to you is sad or having a hard time). What's your magic gift?
- Imagine something you really want to achieve in your life. How will you achieve this?
- If you could invite a historical figure to dinner tonight, who would it be? Why? What would you ask him or her?
- If you could date anyone on earth, past or present, who would it be? Why?
- If you were stranded on a desert island for a year and could pick three CDs and one book, or three books and one CD, what would you choose?
- If you had unlimited funds and a month off starting tomorrow, what would you do?
- What is your slogan/theme song/motto for living life? Explain why, and how it impacts your life.
- What three things are guaranteed to make you smile?
- What song do you love to sing at the top of your lungs? What makes you love it?
- Name something you're scared of but would love to find the guts to do.
- What moment in life gave you goose bumps and why?
- What's something you tried to do but failed? What did you learn by failing?
- Make a wish for each person at the table for something you'd like to see them accomplish this year.
- If you could combine three people on earth (alive or dead, famous or not) to be your perfect mate, who would they be? Why?

I would love to hear from you about your favorite dinner conversation. You can post your favorite conversation-starting questions at www.10daydetox.com/tools.

And, if you want more help turning your dreams into reality, then please visit Coach Lauren's website (www.handelgroup.com) to learn more about how she and her team can help you dream big.

NUTRITION 101: WHAT WE NEVER LEARNED IN SCHOOL

The foundation of your diet should be high-quality protein, fats, and nonstarchy vegetables that don't spike blood sugar or insulin. The reasons are simple: These are the types of foods that not only detoxify your body, reignite your metabolism, calm body-wide inflammation, and crush cravings, but also fill you up. Remember it is very hard to control *how much* you eat, but easy to control *what* you eat. It is the quality of the food and the composition of your meal that matters most in reversing weight gain and creating health.

When you eat the right combination of foods, you can eat until you're gently satisfied without focusing on calories or portion sizes, and excess weight will come off naturally. But since calories have been the focus of conversations around weight loss and health for so long, I'll put it this way: If you eat four Twizzlers—a small amount by most standards—you would consume about 160 calories, and it's unlikely they would put a dent in your hunger. However, for those same 160 calories, you could have a heaping spoonful of almond butter and a practically endless supply of cherry tomatoes, jicama, and celery. I think you'll agree which is the more filling option. Not only that, a snack of nuts helps stabilize your blood sugar and provides you with lots of vitamins, minerals, and phytochemicals—health-protecting substances that ward off diseases such as type 2 diabetes, heart disease, and Alzheimer's disease. The Twizzlers? They have the opposite effect.

Snack foods such as candy bars and other hyperprocessed fare are high on the glycemic index (GI). This is a measure of how quickly a carbohydrate raises your blood sugar level. The index is measured on a scale of

0 to 100, with glucose (a form of simple sugar) having a value of 100. Higher numbers mean that a food causes a sharper rise in blood sugar. It's easy to see why candy would be considered a fast-acting carbohydrate, but you may be surprised to learn that any white flour—white rice, white bread, refined cereals, and even some whole-grain breads—convert to simple sugars in your body quite rapidly. In fact, bread has a higher GI than table sugar or sucrose; 2 slices of whole-wheat bread will raise your blood sugar more than 2 tablespoons of table sugar. On the other hand, nonstarchy vegetables, protein, nuts, seeds, and good fats raise blood sugar levels slowly.

While the glycemic index can be a helpful tool, it doesn't take into account what the rest of your meal looks like, or even how your food is cooked. All of this can impact your blood sugar levels. The best approach to meals is to combine slow-acting carbohydrates—those veggies listed in the produce section on page 41—with lean proteins and healthy fats. In fact, the 10-Day Detox Diet is a high-carb diet—because nonstarchy vegetables, fruits, and even nuts and seeds are all carbs—so it might be more accurate to call it a right-carb diet. You can shift the composition of your diet to help balance your blood sugar, and this will speed up your metabolism, activate burning of belly fat, and cut hunger and cravings. The goal, whether you're eating in your family's dining room, at your work cafeteria, or in a fine restaurant, is to always build your meal from these three types of foods. These three basics—quality proteins, healthy fats, and nonstarchy veggies—can be mixed and matched in any number of ways, so you'll never tire of your options. Have a miso-glazed salmon fillet with pak choi sautéed in avocado oil. Enjoy a spicy chicken breast over a chopped salad with a drizzle of fine olive oil. Dig into a juicy steak served with roasted broccoli and cauliflower. At every meal, you can enjoy a variety of foods, flavors, and textures so you'll never be bored.

Herbs, spices, and seasonings kick your cuisine, and your health, up a notch. Think of your spice cupboard as your new medicine cabinet and stock it with every imaginable seasoning. By flavoring your food liberally, you're not only keeping your taste buds happy, but you're also adding loads of phytonutrients to your meal. Cinnamon, cumin, turmeric, and cayenne pepper—to name just a few—have properties that stabilize blood sugar, quell inflammation, and boost metabolism. Different spices and seasonings have different benefits, which is why I always have lots of these gems on hand. Just be sure to use up your spices often and keep them sealed tightly in jars, as they become less potent with time.

4

Creating a Healing Kitchen

It's quite likely that your kitchen has been held hostage by the food industry. No doubt your cupboards and pantry are filled with ultra-processed fare. Now's your chance to escape these shackles and transform your kitchen into a place of wellness. If you make your kitchen a safe zone, with only foods that nourish rather than harm, then you will automatically make the right choices when it comes time to eat.

Ideally, you're starting the transformation at least two days before you begin your detox. This will give you enough time to clean out your cupboards and fridge, and restock with healing fare.

Start by setting aside at least an hour to scour and purge your pantry, fridge, and freezer. This is your time to do some detective work, read food labels, and dump anything that got you to this food-addicted, toxic state to begin with.

Ideally, your kitchen will mostly showcase foods without labels. Fresh avocados, blueberries, tomatoes, and kiwis don't come in packages and are label-free. But other foods, including nuts, nut butters, almond milk, canned fish, and frozen veggies—foods that I encourage you to eat—do come in packages. Further, once you enter the transition phase, you will be choosing gluten-free grains and other foods that are also minimally processed. It's clear that not *all* packages are bad—and that is why it is so important to get the hang of reading a nutrition facts panel and ingredients list. There is a short learning curve, but once you get the hang of it you will easily spot trouble. Follow these rules when you purchase packaged foods (i.e., anything with a nutrition label):

- **Beware of foods with health claims** on the packaging—such as "reduced sugar" or "no trans fat." These claims usually signal a marketing ploy to make you think the foods are good for you when they're really just pretenders. Things such as sports beverages, energy bars, and even multigrain breads (which often contain high-fructose corn syrup) fall into this category.

- **Focus on the ingredients list.** Remember that the most abundant ingredient is always listed first; the others follow in descending order by weight.

- **Choose foods with fewer than five ingredients** listed, and all things you recognize and know are real food—for example: "tomatoes, water, salt."

- **Buy only packaged foods with ingredients you can pronounce or recognize.** Need to buy something with more than five ingredients? The exception is if they are all whole-food, real ingredients such as spices. The main distinction is that the recipes don't call for things such as "maltodextrin" or "autolyzed yeast extract" or "high-fructose corn syrup." I don't stock these items in my kitchen, and neither should you. Bottom line: You should not eat packaged foods that contain ingredients you wouldn't have in your own kitchen.

- **Be aware that food manufacturers don't have to list ingredients that appear in trace amounts.** These trace ingredients could trip you up in your detox and lifelong quest for eating simple, healthy food. So always be vigilant when selecting multi-ingredient packaged foods. Stick with organic brands, or simple products, or those that declare themselves as gluten- or dairy-free.

- **Avoid these ingredients at all costs** during the 10-Day Detox Diet:
  - **Sugar.** You have to watch for all forms of sugar, not just the word "sugar." There are 257 forms of sugar, most made from corn, with names that you wouldn't recognize, such as maltodextrin and xanthan gum. There are many aliases to watch out for—including organic cane juice, honey, agave, maple syrup,

cane syrup, or molasses. And, look carefully at condiments such as salad dressing, barbecue sauce, or ketchup: There may be up to 33 teaspoons of sugar—often in the form of high-fructose corn syrup—in the average bottle of ketchup (about 1 teaspoon of sugar for every tablespoon of ketchup!). When transitioning off the detox, consider adding sugar back into your diet only as a special treat—to be enjoyed occasionally in small amounts.

- **Other sweeteners** (aspartame, NutraSweet, Splenda, sucralose, and sugar alcohols—any word that ends with "ol," such as xylitol or sorbitol). Stevia may be better than aspartame but only in the form of a whole-plant extract, not Pure Via or Truvia, which are made by Pepsi and Coke and are chemical extracts of stevia. Use it sparingly. A new noncaloric sweetener that comes from monk fruit (also called *luo han guo*) is rich in antioxidants and can also be used in small amounts. But remember, any sweetener can make you hungry, lower your metabolism, create gas, store belly fat, and even change your gut bacteria from those that make you thin to those that make you fat. So it's best to stay away from sweeteners altogether.

- **Bad fats.** Scour labels for the words "hydrogenated fat," just another name for trans fat. As you probably know, the Food and Drug Administration (FDA) has finally declared trans fats not suitable for human consumption. Yet the government has given food companies years to "reformulate" their products, so most processed or packaged foods still contain trans fats...and when there are trace amounts, they are not required to list them. So stay away from industrial, manufactured foodlike substances and science projects.

- **Preservatives, additives, colorings, natural flavorings.** Watch for ingredients you don't recognize or can't pronounce, or that are in Latin. Most of you know that MSG (monosodium glutamate) is a popular taste enhancer, but did you know that it is a brain toxin that causes compulsive overeating and spikes insulin? Knowing this sure makes it easier to avoid this ingredient, doesn't it?

▫ **Dairy.** Because milk is one of the eight most common food allergens, manufacturers are required to clearly identify it on a food label. But casein, the offending protein in dairy, can be found in mayonnaise, chocolate, and "natural" flavors. So be sure to watch for it on the ingredients list.

▫ **Gluten.** Gluten is one of the most common triggers of inflammation in the body and increases cravings and weight gain. It can be lurking in soba noodles, tamari, miso, seasonings, and stock, so look for "gluten-free" listings for these ingredients. But remember, gluten-free cookies are still cookies, and probably contain sugar and other things your body doesn't need.

▫ **Alcohol and caffeine.**

■ **Beware the "Nutrition Facts"** section of the label. Here's why:

▫ **Not the whole story.** A typical nutrition facts label will give you quick stats on cholesterol, fat, carbohydrate, protein, and other nutrients. But, for example, it doesn't differentiate between healthy omega-3 fats and inflammatory omega-6 fats. You can't tell if the quickly absorbed carbs are the bad kind that spike blood sugar or slow-burning, "smart" carbohydrates.

▫ **The "chemical soup" is not on the label.** The "nutrition facts" can't tell you if your food is laced with chemical preservatives, fillers, additives, hormones, antibiotics, pesticides, fertilizers, gluten, dairy, artificial sweeteners, synthetic vitamins, food dyes, and other toxic junk typically present in processed foods. That's why we emphasize paying more attention to the ingredients list and not spending too much time on the nutrition facts label.

▫ **Focus on fiber, sugar, and protein per serving.** These three facts will help you discern whether the food can help regulate your blood sugars or send them skyrocketing.

　■ Keep total sugars less than 8 grams per meal.

　■ Aim to include at least 5 to 10 grams of fiber with every meal.

　■ Aim for a minimum of 10 grams of protein with every meal, but up to 30 or 40 grams is fine. Include protein with every meal because it keeps your blood sugars stable, prevents cravings, and builds fat-blasting muscle. For more information on what amount of protein and nutrition is appropriate for you, please visit my online nutrition team at www.10daydetox .com/tools.

- **Serving size.** Look at this carefully to determine whether this is your "typical" portion, as labels can be deceiving. For example, a 20-ounce soda says "2.5 servings," but do you usually share your soda with 1.5 other people? All of the stats on the panel are related to serving size, so once you determine how much you eat, you can figure out how much of each nutrient you'll be getting.

- **Fats** are broken down by type. On most labels you will find total fat, saturated fat, and trans fat. Some labels of foods rich in fat (oil, for example) will also tell you how much monounsaturated and polyunsaturated fats you are getting. If your label shows only the former three, you can subtract the saturated and trans fat from the total fat content in order to know how many grams of mono- and polyunsaturated fats you are getting. Monounsaturated and omega-3 polyunsaturated fats should dominate this category. Saturated fats are turning out not to be the bad guys we thought they were. While they do raise LDL, they also increase HDL and good fluffy cholesterol particles. In fact, in a recent review of 72 studies, there was no correlation between fat — even saturated fat — and heart disease. You want to look for zero trans fats. But be careful: If a serving has less than 0.5 gram of trans fat, the nutrition facts label can legally say "zero trans fats." Processed whipped cream, for instance, says it contains zero trans fats, but the three main ingredients are water, hydrogenated vegetable oil (another term for trans fats), and high-fructose corn syrup.

- **Total carbohydrates** include the amount of sugar (whether naturally occurring or added during processing) as well as fiber. This gives you a picture of how the food will impact your blood sugar. Think of fiber as the drain stopper of your stomach. Fiber slows the rate at which sugar from your food enters your bloodstream from your intestines. So, the more fiber a food contains, the slower your blood sugar will rise upon eating it. If you don't currently eat a high-fiber diet, start adding fiber slowly so that you don't cause any digestive distress. Your ultimate goal should be to consume around 50 grams daily. That may sound like a lot, but if you eat according to the guidelines outlined in this book, you will have no problem achieving that. Remember that foods that are naturally low in sugar (less than 10 grams) and high in fiber (more than 5 grams) are slow-acting carbohydrates, the kind you want.

◻ **Fiber** is one of the main factors that determine how slowly (or quickly) a carbohydrate enters your bloodstream. Most of the packaged foods you'll be eating—such as nuts and frozen vegetables—are naturally rich in fiber. Some packaged foods, however, have added fibers. One type of fiber is called resistant starch because it escapes digestion in your small intestine. The fact is, you don't know what you are getting when you see this, and for all you know it could be sawdust! (Some bread makers actually use sawdust as a resistant starch to lower the net carbs of the bread.) Putting sawdust in food doesn't make it healthy; eating real forms of fiber such as vegetables, seeds, and nuts is healthy. Stay away from any type of fiber that is not naturally a part of your food. In fact, for the most part, if you see a fiber in the ingredients list, you know this product is better for the company's marketing department than your body! There are many ways to tell if a food product is good or lousy. If a manufacturer is bragging about the fiber content of a certain food, there's a good chance that fiber has been added in the form of inulin (also known as oligofructose or chicory root fiber), polydextrose, resistant starch, or wheat dextrin. Always scan the ingredients list to look for these terms and avoid foods made with them. Stick with whole-food fiber, not sawdust or engineered forms of fiber.

◻ **Cholesterol** in foods is not the problem we once thought it was. There is little correlation between dietary cholesterol and blood cholesterol, and little reason to worry about this number on food labels. Surprising but true.

▫ **Sodium** is abundant in packaged foods. As much as 70 percent of the sodium in your diet could be coming from packaged food sold in your supermarket. Companies add sodium to give packaged foods flavor, but fresh foods don't need much salt to taste fabulous. When you eat whole foods, you naturally get the right amount of sodium your body needs. By following my program, you will easily cut down on and normalize your sodium intake. Current dietary guidelines suggest to keep sodium intake under 2,300 milligrams. Yet, new research shows that the lowest risk of mortality comes from an intake of 3,000 to 6,000 milligrams per day. Interestingly, Japanese people consume an average of 4,500 milligrams of sodium per day and have one of the highest life expectancies in the world, with low cardiovascular risk. What does all this mean? Sodium itself is not the culprit, but an unhealthy diet full of processed foods, inflammatory fats, and refined carbohydrates is. When you don't include fresh, real food—namely, potassium-rich vegetables and low-glycemic fruits—you increase your sodium-to-potassium ratio. Because potassium helps you excrete fluid, it helps to relieve the pressure in your circulatory system. If you consume too much sodium, as is the case when you eat a processed foods–based diet, your blood pressure may rise, especially if you have diabesity. The goal is to include plenty of potassium-rich foods and crowd out the sodium-rich processed junk. When you cook meals at home with these recipes you will learn how to add the right amount and type of salt to flavor your food and nourish your body. Play around with adding real flavor to your meals by using tasty seasonings such as curry powder, chili peppers, rosemary, sage, and cinnamon. The less salt you add, the less you will want, as your taste buds will adapt to your new eating habits.

▫ **Protein** is your secret weapon to success on this program because it reduces insulin spikes and keeps you feeling satisfied long after you've eaten. Each protein is made of specific amino acids. Amino acids are the building blocks of protein and are either essential or nonessential. Essential amino acids cannot be produced in the body and need to be consumed through diet, while nonessential amino acids can be produced in the body from other sources of carbohydrates or proteins. When we consume animal protein or soy protein, we ensure that our body receives complete, high-biological-value protein. This is important for detoxifying and getting and maintaining health. Remember that diversity is the key to nutrition, so eat a variety of whole foods to meet your protein needs. Opt for protein sources such as high-quality meat, clean fish, poultry, omega 3–enriched eggs, tofu, and nuts.

- **Vitamins and minerals** are listed at the bottom of the nutrition facts panel, but eyeball these with caution. Sometimes junk foods are fortified with nutrients to enhance their appeal. For example, B vitamins are added to foods to "enrich" them, but that is only because they are impoverished in the first place. Obviously, a food put together from various artificial ingredients won't naturally contain the valuable nutrients you would get if you just ate the real thing. Take vitamin water, for example. It is a farce, a brilliant marketing ploy for one more type of sugar water sold by Coke. We all know that water doesn't naturally contain vitamins! And candy, too—do you really think gummy bears have naturally occurring vitamin C? Look at this part of the food panel carefully and you'll be able to sort out good food from junk food.

- **Stay away from "foodlike substances."** These are things that, through processing, no longer resemble the real food in its true form. Veggie burgers made with soy protein isolates—a cheap form of processed soy—are a hijacked version of soy in its whole form (for example, tofu).

Knowing what to avoid is important. However, you are probably wondering about everything that is in your pantry and refrigerator right now. What's okay and not okay to use during the detox? What should I avoid and then safely reintroduce? Here's a general guide to the items that should be tossed out permanently or put aside for the next ten days.

ITEMS THAT NEED TO GO PERMANENTLY:

- Highly refined cooking oils such as corn and soy.
- Fried foods you may have stored in your freezer.
- Margarine or shortening, which contain those dreaded hydrogenated fats we discussed earlier.

ITEMS THAT SHOULD BE AVOIDED FOR THE NEXT TEN DAYS (find a spot for them where they are out of sight, as you may choose to reintroduce these in your transition phase):

- All gluten-containing products (including whole-grain versions), such as pasta, bread, and cereal.
- All grains (including gluten-free versions), such as quinoa and rice.
- All dairy products (including but not limited to butter, milk, yogurt, and cheese—from any animal).
- All beans (including chickpeas, lentils, and even peanuts, which are actually beans).
- Any prepared food that was made in your local store or by a small manufacturer. It's best to steer clear of premade foods altogether because certain items might be left off the ingredients list due to FDA labeling guidelines.
- All alcohol, as it is simply sugar in a different form, and it impairs impulse control so you're more likely to eat more—and to do so mindlessly. It also has more calories per gram than sugar (7 calories compared to 4 calories), provokes a leaky gut, and inflames your liver. While it is not all about the calories, if you have one glass of wine a day at 110 calories, over the course of a year that can add up to 11 pounds (5 kg) of weight gain.
- Caffeine. Some say caffeine speeds up metabolism or the rate of calorie burning, called *thermogenesis*. But so do spicy jalapeños or cayenne pepper. Caffeine is hidden in many soft drinks and energy

drinks because it is addictive, so you consume more of the sugary drinks. Caffeine also increases hunger.

Now that you've cleaned out your kitchen, you will automatically steer clear of the toxic foods that cause addiction, weight problems, and health struggles. Consider yourself liberated!

STOCKING YOUR KITCHEN WITH WHAT YOU *CAN* EAT — MY GUIDE TO LIVING CLEAN AND GREEN

Now that there's all that room in your fridge and cabinets, let's have some fun filling them up with real, fresh food. This is where we begin to discover all the amazing new options you have. Perhaps it's been a while since you explored the produce section of your grocery store or visited a farmers' market. Maybe you're unfamiliar with the bounty of fresh vegetables that you can use as the basis for many meals at the foundation of this program. The key to success is a well-stocked kitchen, which allows you to whip up a meal on even the busiest of days.

I am proud to be on the board of directors for the Environmental Working Group (EWG) because what we do to our bodies we do to the planet, and what we do to the planet we do to our bodies. The link between environmental toxins and chronic disease is now clear. We know that pesticides and other industrial chemicals cause obesity and type 2 diabetes. There is a new word for these compounds: *obesogens*. When we are toxic, we feel lousy, gain unwanted pounds, and have trouble losing them. Toxins disrupt the hormones that regulate our metabolism.

The recipes in this book will help you live clean and green by using foods that contain special phytochemicals that increase your body's capacity for detoxification and balance your blood sugar. They are designed to put your medicine on the end of your fork.

Here are some of the fresh and pantry food items you should always have on hand.

Produce

Fresh vegetables and fruits make up half of all of my meals. But before we go crazy buying just any produce, I'd like to talk a little bit about making the right selections. Agricultural chemical inputs such as pesticides and fertilizers leave a residue, which we as consumers absorb. Because these chemicals are fat-soluble, they become stored in our fat cells. Our bodies recognize these toxins as foreign, prompting an inflammatory response. Once our exposure surpasses our threshold, we become sick and fat.

When you can, avoid the most pesticide-contaminated fruits and vegetables. The EWG annually reviews conventional vegetables and fruits and publishes a list of those with the lowest and highest toxic load. EWG understands that we have a right to know which foods are safe and which we need to be concerned about. They provide many resources for consumers, including their Shopper's Guide, which helps consumers opt out of the produce posing the highest risk while saving their food dollars for the safer choices. For an easier reference, check out their "Dirty Dozen" and "Clean Fifteen" lists featuring the most- and least-contaminated options in the conventional food supply. Of course, you can still buy items from the "Dirty Dozen" list, but they should be organic. As of the date of publication of this book, these are featured below. To make the most informed choices for you and your loved ones, visit EWG's website at www.ewg.org for the most updated lists.

THE DIRTY DOZEN:

1. Apples
2. Strawberries
3. Grapes
4. Celery
5. Peaches
6. Spinach
7. Sweet peppers
8. Imported nectarines
9. Cucumbers

10. Cherry tomatoes
11. Imported sugar snap peas
12. Potatoes

THE CLEAN FIFTEEN:

1. Avocados
2. Sweetcorn
3. Pineapples
4. Cabbage
5. Frozen peas
6. Onions
7. Asparagus
8. Mangoes
9. Papayas
10. Kiwis
11. Aubergines
12. Grapefruit
13. Melon
14. Cauliflower
15. Sweet potatoes

WHAT TO STOCK UP ON

- When possible, choose organic, seasonal, local produce. Be sure to check out your local farmers' market or community-supported agriculture (CSA) group.
- For those living in colder climates, you can find organic versions of your favorite fruits and vegetables in the freezer section. Always make sure you're buying unseasoned or unsweetened varieties.
- Nonstarchy veggies are freebies—eat as many as you like! A limited selection of fruits are included on this plan because most fruits increase your insulin levels. I have included those fruits that support you with the right vitamins, minerals, and antioxidants. Following is a list of low-GI, low-sugar vegetables and fruits you can eat while on this program. Many of them are incorporated into the

delicious recipes in the pages ahead. If you have a few favorites that appear on this list but don't appear in the recipes, feel free to substitute them at any time.

- Artichokes
- Asparagus
- Aubergine
- Avocados
- Bean sprouts
- Beet greens
- Blueberries
- Broccoli
- Brussels sprouts
- Cabbage
- Cauliflower
- Celery
- Chicory
- Chives
- Courgettes
- Dandelion greens
- Fennel
- Fresh herbs
- Garlic
- Ginger
- Green beans
- Hearts of palm
- Jalapeño chilies
- Kale
- Kiwis
- Lemons
- Lettuce
- Limes
- Mangetout
- Mushrooms
- Mustard greens
- Onions
- Peppers
- Pomegranate seeds
- Radicchio
- Radishes
- Rocket
- Shallots
- Spinach
- Spring greens
- Sugar snap peas
- Swiss chard
- Tomatoes
- Watercress

Fresh Meats and Proteins

What about meat, poultry, fish, and eggs? As best you can, limit your exposure to excessive hormones, antibiotics, and grain-fed meat. Select wild meat, grass-fed when possible, and organic poultry and eggs. Because we eat what the animal ate, we want our animal-based protein to have been fed the highest-quality diet. An animal fed its natural diet, typically grass and plants, contains fewer stress hormones, growth hormones, and antibiotics than an intensively reared animal on industrially produced animal foods. By selecting higher-quality animal-based proteins, you can be sure you are getting healthier fats and leaner, cleaner protein.

When it comes to selecting poultry, the U.S. Department of Agriculture (USDA) mandates that all poultry be raised without the use of hormones. However, chicken producers must give medications to those birds that get sick before selling them. Therefore, always look for the terms "antibiotic-free" or "organic" when buying poultry to ensure you are truly getting a toxin-free product.

Get in the habit of keeping your fridge and freezer stocked with the items below:

- Grass-fed, hormone-free, or organic beef, lamb, and bison (buffalo) meat (refer to the Environmental Working Group's "Meat Eater's Guide" at www.ewg.org to choose meat that's good for you and good for the planet).
- Organic or antibiotic-free boneless, skinless chicken and turkey breasts and minced chicken and turkey.
- Wild or sustainably farmed low-mercury seafood such as clams, crab, herring, oyster, perch, plaice, pollock, salmon, sardines, shrimp, sole, squid and trout. Avoid fish that are high in mercury, such as tuna, swordfish, and Chilean sea bass. Go to the Marine Stewardship Council website (www.MSC.org) and download their Sustainable Seafood Guide to choosing the fish lowest in mercury.
- Organic omega 3–enriched eggs.
- Organic, whole forms of non-GMO (genetically modified organisms) soy food, such as tofu, tempeh, and gluten-free, low-sodium miso.

With these healthy pantry staples in your cooking arsenal, you'll be amazed at the delicious and nutritious dishes you can create. Cooking food that tastes great and nourishes your body doesn't need to break the bank, either—and that's why I stock my pantry with food from Thrive Market, an online organic food retailer.

Healing Pantry Staples

The recipes in this book celebrate real, whole, fresh food. They are easily made in your kitchen yet taste as if they came from a restaurant. We live in a food desert, so our reliance on getting back into the kitchen to enjoy a meal that is both satisfying and healthy requires us to learn how to cook again. The following are some of the ingredients I use the most in my own kitchen :

- Extra-virgin olive oil
- Extra-virgin coconut butter/oil (at room temperature it is solid, but it melts into a liquid)
- Other healthy oils, such as walnut, sesame, grapeseed, flax, or avocado
- Nut butters (raw, if possible), such as almond, cashew, macadamia, or walnut
- Nuts, such as walnuts, almonds, pecans, and macadamias
- Seeds, such as hemp, chia, flax, pumpkin, and sesame
- Tahini (sesame seed paste)
- Full-fat unsweetened coconut milk
- Unsweetened hemp or almond milk
- Canned or jarred Kalamata olives
- Almond flour (also called almond meal)
- Arrowroot
- Apple cider vinegar
- Balsamic vinegar
- Gluten-free, low-sodium tamari
- Low-sodium vegetable or chicken stock
- Dijon mustard
- Sea salt
- Black peppercorns (for grinding)
- Dried herbs and spices, such as basil, cayenne pepper, chili powder, cinnamon, coriander, cumin, onion powder, oregano, paprika, parsley, rosemary, sage, thyme, turmeric

Some of the items listed above may be familiar to you and others not so much. Whether you are new to cooking or just to learning how to cook healthy options, I want to introduce you to some amazing ingredients that can enhance your meals and provide some variety:

Almond Flour

Made from blanched and finely ground almonds, almond flour (also known as almond meal) is a low-glycemic alternative to grain-based flours such as wheat flour. Use almond flour in place of gluten-based flours when making muffins, breads, or other baked goods.

Arrowroot

During the 10-Day Detox Diet, all grains, including corn, need to be omitted from your meal plan. Arrowroot is a corn-free, hypoallergenic alternative to cornflour. Remember, corn in any form is still a grain and a potential allergen. Arrowroot is a useful culinary tool for your sauces or stews.

Chia Seeds

Chia seeds are one of the few vegetarian and vegan sources of omega-3 fatty acids. When they absorb water, they gel into a pudding-like substance that adds great texture to shakes, desserts, and cereals.

Coconut Aminos

If you are soy-intolerant, try using a little coconut aminos for that soy sauce flavor. It is made from the sap of the palm tree and imparts a slightly sweet aftertaste. Coconut aminos are rich in amino acids—the building blocks of protein.

Coconut Butter

I use coconut butter to add a silky texture and buttery flavor to morning shakes. It is made from whole coconut flesh, not just the oil. The butter provides fiber, protein, and nutrients to help keep you satisfied. Coconut butter can be found in most grocery stores near the other nut and seed butters.

Coconut Cream

When you remove excess water from coconut milk and strain it, you are left with a rich cream that is slightly sweet and full of healthy fat. It is a great alternative to dairy cream—a little bit goes a long way.

Coconut Flour

Coconut flour is a nutty, slightly sweet alternative to grain-based flours. Unlike wheat flour, coconut flour is not heavily refined, so most of its nutrition remains intact. Dried coconut meat is defatted and ground to a granular texture. It is useful in baked products and often found in grain-free cereals. High in fiber and very low in carbohydrates, it is a great tool in your detox kitchen.

Coconut Milk

The slightly sweet flavor of coconut milk makes it a healthy alternative to dairy milk. It is rich in saturated fat and healthy medium-chain triglycerides, which studies show boost metabolism and have other health benefits. You can buy whole-fat organic canned coconut milk and mix it with four cans of water to create your own coconut milk without sweeteners or stabilizers.

Coconut Oil

Coconut oil is extracted from the whole coconut, and unlike coconut butter, the oil does not contain fiber or protein. Studies have shown that coconut oil, used in sautés, shakes, sauces, or baking, helps improve blood sugar regulation, boosts immunity, and even increases the ratio of HDL to LDL cholesterol so you have more healthy lipids in your circulation. Look for whole-kernel, expeller-pressed coconut oil to get the most benefits.

Flaxseed Meal

Flaxseed meal is a nutrition powerhouse and a great vegetarian source of omega-3 fatty acids, lignans, and fiber. Add a tablespoon or two to shakes to add fiber and promote healthy elimination. Use freshly ground flax-seed meal when possible, and store it in your refrigerator.

Grapeseed Oil

Grapeseed oil is extracted from the seeds of grapes. It has a healthy fat profile of monounsaturated and polyunsaturated fats. I use it for higher-heat cooking and baking as it has a higher smoke point (the point at which an oil smokes and becomes rancid). Because it has a neutral flavor, you can use it as a healthier alternative to rapeseed oil.

Hemp Protein Powder

Hemp protein powder is a hypoallergenic plant-based protein that can boost the protein content of your morning shakes or smoothies. Look for unsweetened protein powders. Sometimes hemp protein is combined with chia, rice, or pea proteins for a vegetarian or vegan protein blend with a smooth texture.

Hemp Seed

Hemp seed is an excellent complete protein as it contains all nine essential amino acids as well as essential fatty acids such as omega-3 fats. It has an earthy, nutty flavor, which balances the sweetness of berries in your morning shakes. Enjoy it in smoothies, nut and seed mixes, or even baked on chicken.

Kelp Noodles

Kelp noodles are made from the sea vegetable. They are simple to pre-pare, eaten raw, and low in carbohydrates. Their neutral flavor makes them fun to include in meals containing sauces such as curries or in broths such as miso soup.

Mayonnaise

Real mayo, made from omega 3–enriched eggs, is simple to make and adds an indulgence to your snacks and sauces. I've included a recipe (page 299) so you can avoid the unhealthy soybean oils, preservatives, and sugar in store-bought mayo.

Miso

Miso adds a deep, comforting element to dishes and intensifies the overall flavor. There are various kinds of miso, ranging from white and yellow, which tend to be mild, to red, brown, and even black miso. Generally, the deeper the color, the longer the miso has fermented and the stronger the taste. Mild miso tastes less salty, and stronger miso offers more of that umami, or savory, salty taste. Some miso pastes have been fermented with grains, especially gluten grains such as barley. Be sure to use miso that has only soybeans, water, and salt on the ingredients list. Brown miso, such as *hatcho,* is gluten-free and contains only fermented soybeans.

Mustard

Mustard, made from ground mustard seeds, is rich in antioxidants and other detox-friendly phytonutrients. Mustard is a lovely complement to any fish, chicken, or meat. It is also delicious in homemade dressings, marinades, and sauces.

Palm Shortening

Palm shortening, made from palm oil, is a great alternative to hydrogenated oils traditionally used in shortening. I like it because it has 0 trans fats and is gluten- and dairy-free. You'll find that it works well in baking because it has a neutral flavor and adds that tasty, fatty mouth feel you are used to enjoying in baked goods.

Sea Salt

When you eat real food and not overly salted processed food, you can use more salt. While seafood, meat, and some vegetables are naturally rich in sodium, you can still enjoy flavoring your meals with moderate quantities of real sea salt. Avoid table salt, which is refined and devoid of sulfur, zinc, iron, calcium, potassium, and magnesium, which naturally occur in sea salt.

Seaweed

Vegetables from the sea, such as dulse, wakame, nori, and kombu, are dense in minerals and vitamins such as potassium, calcium, iron, magnesium, iodine, and selenium. Use seaweed in salads, soups, and stews to add a hint of savory.

Shirataki Noodles

Traditionally made with konjac root, these low-glycemic noodles are gluten- (and guilt-) free.

Tamari

Look for gluten-free, low-sodium tamari for a healthier alternative to soy sauce.

Thai Fish Sauce

Fish sauce has a complex flavor that complements the sweet flavors of traditional Thai cooking. I love using a dash of fish sauce to impress dinner guests. It adds that wow factor that will leave your guests wondering how you learned to cook so well!

Replace This with That

For the next ten days, you're challenged with a radical change in the way you've been eating. My bet is that after the ten days are up, you'll want to stick to many of the principles of the basic plan. Once you get into the transition phase, you can start to gradually add in other foods, depending on how much weight you still need to lose and your personal health goals. I offer the following suggestions to help you adapt to this way of life, but feel free to get creative in the kitchen to find substitutions that help you stay on track.

INSTEAD OF	TRY
Fruit-flavored yogurt	Chia pudding
Pasta	Shirataki noodles
Mashed potatoes	Cauliflower mash
Rice	Cauliflower "rice"
Peanut butter	Almond or other nut butters
Potato crisps, pretzels, tortilla chips	Nuts
Parmesan cheese	Nutritional yeast
Cornflour	Arrowroot
Dairy milk	Unsweetened coconut milk or almond milk
Canned tuna	Canned wild salmon
Butter	Coconut oil or butter
Wheat flour	Almond flour or coconut flour
Bread, wraps, or buns	Round or romaine lettuce leaves
Milk chocolate	Raw cacao or 75% dark chocolate

5

Tips and Tools

Now that we have discussed the facts behind making the right choices, identified the good and the bad, and helped you restock your kitchen for success, I'd like to provide you with some quick tips to make the next ten days—and the rest of your life—a little easier. Change and transition are not easy, so hopefully the information on the next few pages will be useful.

KITCHEN TOOL ESSENTIALS

Would you set out to begin a DIY project without a hammer or other necessary equipment? Of course not! If you want to cook you need a well-stocked kitchen. I suggest you have the following tools on hand—they'll make cooking fast, simple, and fun.

- a set of good-quality knives
- two wooden chopping boards—one for animal products, another for fruits and vegetables
- a 20-cm and a 30-cm nonstick (non-Teflon) sauté pan
- an 8-liter stockpot
- a 2-liter and a 4-liter saucepan with lids
- a 27-cm-square nonstick (non-Teflon) griddle pan
- a cast-iron casserole
- several rimmed baking sheets

- several square and/or rectangular baking dishes
- a food processor
- a blender
- a stick blender
- an instant-read thermometer
- a coffee grinder for flaxseed and spices
- wire whisks
- spring tongs
- a fish spatula
- rubber spatulas
- a vegetable steaming rack or basket
- glass measuring jug
- assorted measuring spoons
- a citrus reamer
- Microplane graters/zesters in assorted sizes
- a food mill
- natural baking paper and foil
- a timer
- sealable glass containers in various sizes for storing leftovers (plastic contains known hormone disruptors, which have been associated with insulin resistance and weight gain as well as female hormonal imbalance and thyroid disease)

SHORTCUTS AND TIME SAVERS

One question I am often asked is: How do I detox on a busy schedule? Trust me, it's easier than you think, but it does require a little planning. I find that when I invest that time, it pays off by keeping me healthy and eating well. In the end, it makes life a little easier, too. Here are some of my own recommended time savers:

- Cook once and eat twice by doubling the recipe and enjoying leftovers later in the week.

- Do as much prep work as possible the night before you plan to cook.
- Chop veggies ahead of time and store them in airtight containers, ready to be used in salads, stir-fries, and other recipes. Precut produce is also available at many supermarkets, both in bags in the produce aisle and at the salad bar. Although it may be a bit more expensive, it drastically reduces prep work.
- Frozen vegetables (preferably organic) are a real time-saver—especially if you already have some in your freezer and can avoid the need for last-minute shopping stops. Some store brands provide high-quality, organic frozen vegetables that were picked and flash-frozen at the peak of freshness.
- Choose fresh prewashed organic leafy greens, such as spinach, kale, rocket, and romaine lettuce.
- Make sauces and marinades and, if you're in the transition phase, cook brown rice and other whole grains in advance.
- Carefully chosen canned and jarred foods, such as vegetable or chicken stock, sardines, wild Alaskan salmon, artichoke hearts, and roasted red peppers, make it easy to toss together last-minute meals and enhance salads. Remember to choose low-sodium versions and read labels carefully to avoid gluten, dairy, sugars, and other unwanted ingredients.
- Choose two days during the week (Sunday and Wednesday seem to work well for many people) when you are going to spend a few extra hours in the kitchen, cooking and preparing as much as you can in advance. With all of your ingredients ready to go, a fresh home-cooked meal can be on the table in less time than it takes the take-out delivery to reach your home.

PLAN YOUR MEALS, SHOP, AND PREPARE FOOD IN ADVANCE

Let's face it: If you wait to decide what to eat until just before you leave for work or just after you get home in the evening, you may not have everything you need to put a meal on the table. Being caught off-guard while having a growling tummy could put you in danger of going off the program entirely and just grabbing what is available, quick, and easy—usually addictive, processed junk. That's where planning comes in. Take some time one day per week to sit down and plan your meals for the upcoming week, and make a shopping list. Go to the grocery store and purchase all of the ingredients for those recipes in advance. Make sure to stick a few frozen goodies in your cart—such as frozen produce or prawns—which will come in handy as you work your way through the fresh food earlier in the week.

Remember, no matter how challenging the prep work seems at first, I promise you'll find that it gets easier and easier, and you'll be a whiz at planning meals in no time. You'll come to appreciate arriving home to a fridge filled with marinated meat and chopped veggies just waiting to be stir-fried.

I totally understand the instinct to order takeout when you're tired after a long day of work. But if you want to detoxify your body, calm the inflammation that's ravaging your system, balance your hormones, lose weight, and reverse diabesity, it's crucial to stick to the plan.

GOOD FOOD ON A TIGHT BUDGET

Relying on inexpensive, overly processed food is tempting, given our demanding lives and schedules, but the cost is actually much greater than it appears. Feasting on salt, fat, and sugar can lead to serious diseases that cost hundreds of dollars in doctor's visits and prescription drugs. We can become sick and sluggish, resulting in less productivity. We might have less patience for our loved ones and less energy to work or enjoy ourselves. Considering the real cost of cheap, processed food, you can't afford *not* to cook.

By now some of you might be wondering how to make this work on your budget. It helps to track all of your expenses for one week and see how much of what you spent went toward achieving your health goals. Right off the bat, you'll be able to spot recurring items and pricey habits that don't get you closer to your goals. For example, if you brew your own coffee each day instead of stopping at a coffee shop, you could save up to £1,000 a year. Do you order takeout for office lunches and Friday night dinners? You may be surprised to find that cooking your own food—even the high-quality food I'm talking about—can save you money. By reorganizing your budget and taking a look at other nonessential discretionary spending, you might create more funding for good food.

You can continue to save money even after you adjust your budget. I recommend getting a copy of "Good Food on a Tight Budget" by the Environmental Working Group (www.ewg.org) to learn what foods are good for you, good for the planet, and good for your wallet. Stick with simple ingredients and a handful of spices that you can use in many dishes, rather than expensive ingredients that you'd use less often. Shop at discount stores or shopping clubs like Costco. Get fresh, local produce from a community-supported agriculture (CSA) group or farmers' market. Look at store circulars to see what's on sale, and shop private-label brands, many of which offer high-quality, organic staple items.

HEALTHY SNACKING

My version of detox doesn't involve juicing, fasting, or even hunger. You'll find that when you eat real, nutritious foods, you will be naturally satisfied. That said, if you go too long between meals or find that you are hungry outside of mealtimes, it helps to have a snack on hand.

For many, however, snacking has become reckless behavior, synonymous with eating a candy bar from a vending machine or nibbling through a bag of crisps, a carton of cookies, or some other salty or sweet packaged item. Let's recast how you think about snacking so you can change your habits.

If you eat well and keep your blood sugar balanced according to the principles of the 10-Day Detox Diet, you probably won't need a snack. But sometimes you might. I view snacking as another occasion to flood your system with protective nutrients that quell hunger, quiet inflammation, and steady your blood sugar. Just as you do at meals, you should combine nonstarchy veggies with quality proteins and healthy fats for

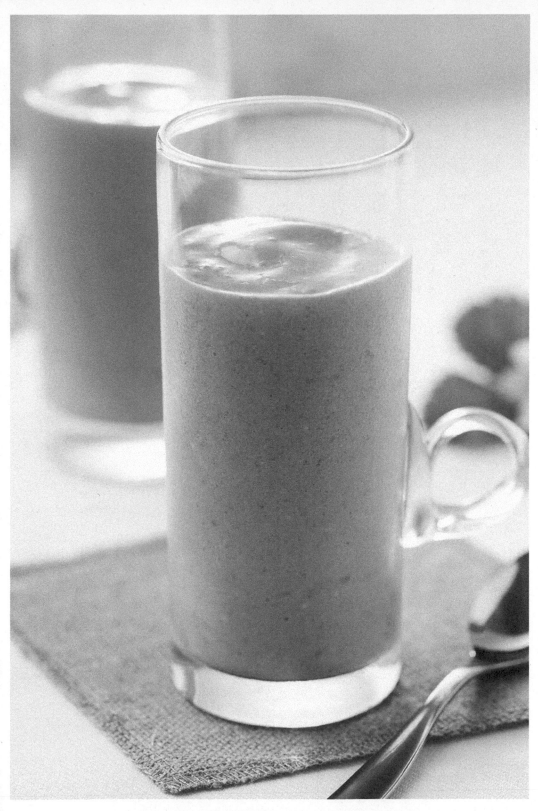

Creamy Berry Smoothie (page 67)

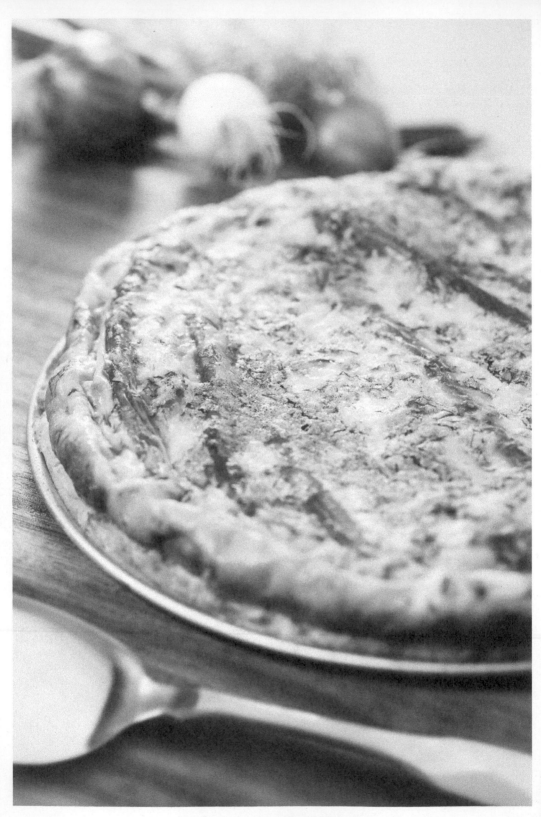

Crustless Asparagus Quiche (page 70)

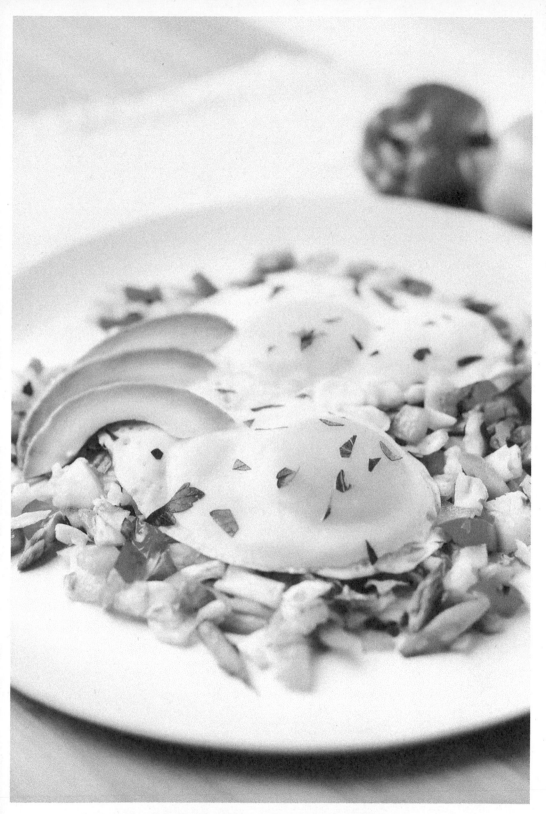

Vegetable Hash with Fried Eggs (page 71)

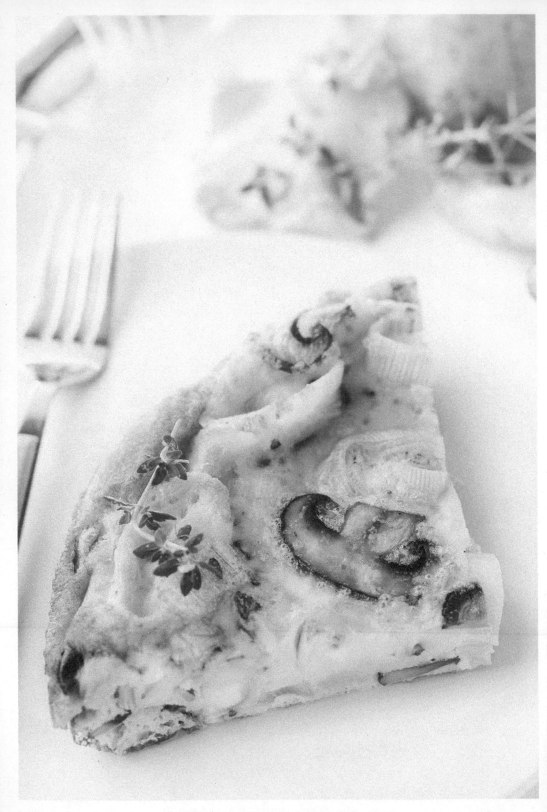

Wild Mushroom and Leek Frittata (page 77)

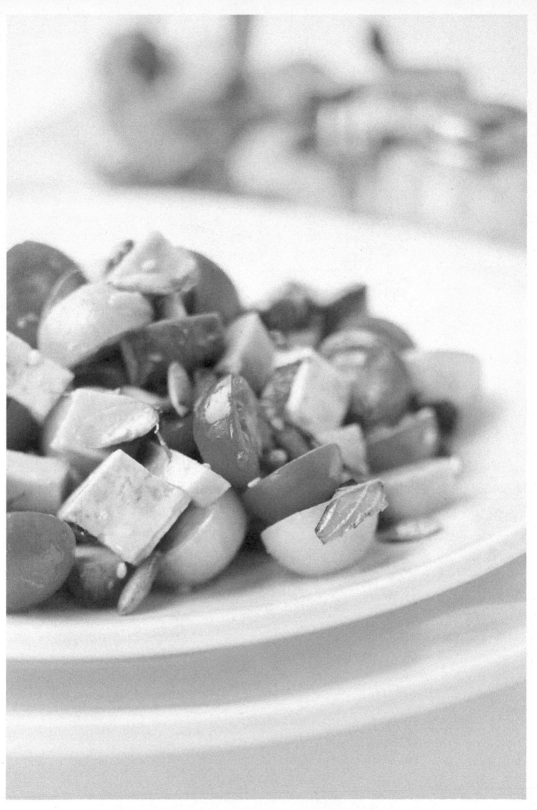

Cherry Tomato and Tofu Salad (page 89)

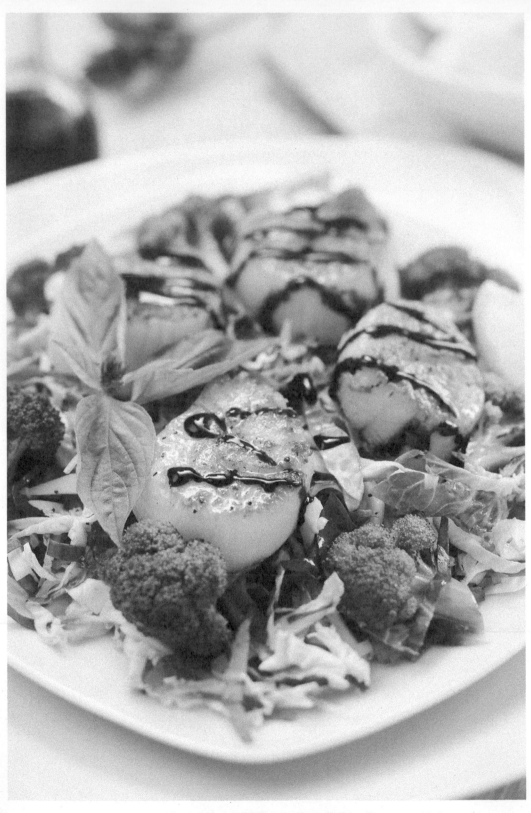

Brussels Sprouts and Broccoli Slaw with Seared Scallops (page 91)

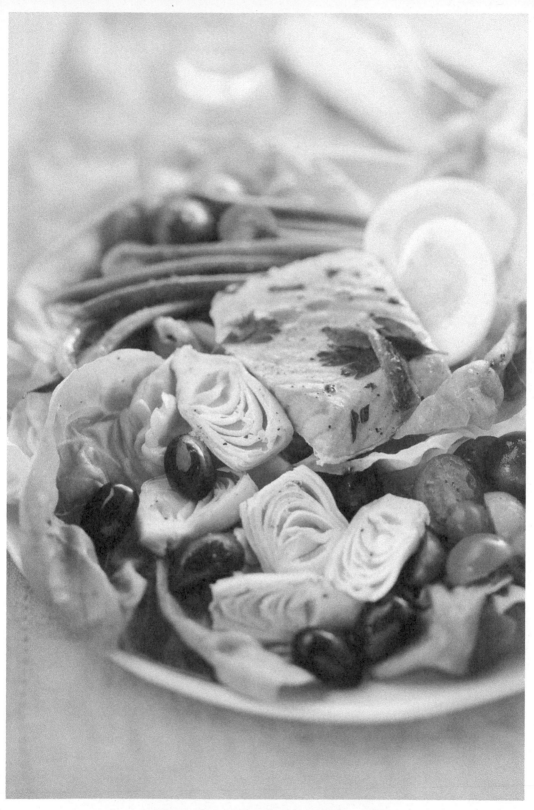

Niçoise Salad with Poached Salmon (page 100)

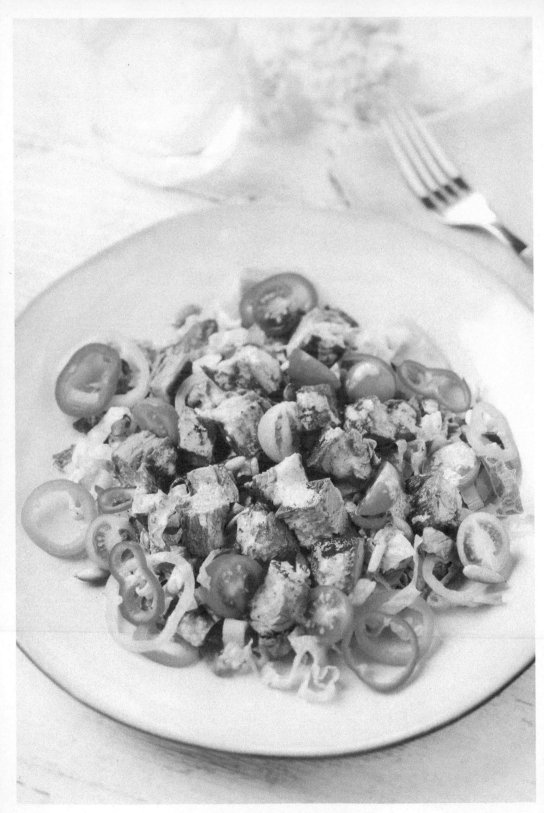

Taco Salad with Skirt Steak (page 124)

snacks. There are many flavorful ways to do this: Enjoy celery sticks with almond butter, a "mezze" plate with a variety of nuts and vegetables, a slice of natural deli meat (without nitrates, high-fructose corn syrup, or preservatives) spread with mashed avocado and wrapped around a romaine leaf, or a hardboiled egg with sliced red pepper. The beauty of the program is that you can be completely flexible once you get used to a few simple guidelines.

Although I don't believe in counting calories or policing portion sizes, your between-meal eating occasions should be smaller than your regular meals. Eat until you are comfortably satisfied, and there's a good chance you're eating the right amount. The key is to keep a variety of healthy snacks on hand so that you're not tempted to visit the vending machine when your stomach starts to growl.

6

How to Prepare Simple Meals

While you'll find that many of the recipes in this cookbook come together quickly and easily, I know that sometimes you are absolutely stuck for time. So, rather than go for the quick-and-dirty takeout option, check out this guide to putting together easy meals using just a few simple ingredients.

COOKING VEGETABLES

Steaming or sautéing veggies takes very little time — especially if you start with precut produce.

To Steam:

Pour 250 ml water in the bottom of a saucepan and bring it to the boil over high heat. Place a steaming rack or basket over the boiling water.

Chop your veggies (or use precut ones), place them in the steaming rack, cover, and steam them for 4 to 8 minutes, depending on the vegetable and your desired level of tenderness. They should still be crunchy, as overcooked vegetables are mushy and less nutritious.

Add your favorite seasonings, drizzle with extra-virgin olive oil, and sprinkle with a little sea salt and freshly ground black pepper to taste. You can cook almost any vegetable this way, and both prep and cleanup are a breeze.

To Sauté:

Heat 1 tablespoon extra-virgin olive oil or other favorite oil, such as coconut oil, in a sauté pan over medium-high heat.

Chop your veggies (or use pre-cut ones) and drop them in. Sauté to your desired flavor and tenderness, 5 to 7 minutes.

Onions, garlic, and/or mushrooms are tasty additions to sautéed veggies. Not only do they make them more flavorful and fragrant, they also boost the phytonutrient content. You might want to sauté these first with a little salt before adding the chopped veggies. Add spices for extra flavor and healing power.

COOKING FISH, CHICKEN, AND MEAT

Fish, chicken, and meat are simple to prepare in a delicious and healthy way. Just grill or sauté, then season with olive oil, lemon juice, rosemary, garlic, ginger, and/or coriander. Another easy flavor-enhancer and nutrient-booster is dairy-free pesto. See page 293 for a simple recipe—it will keep for months in your freezer, so you can make a big batch.

To Grill:

Preheat the grill or a griddle pan. Sprinkle sea salt, freshly ground black pepper, and any other seasonings you like on your fish fillets or steaks; boneless, skinless chicken breasts; or lean cuts of meat. If you use spice blends, make sure they don't contain MSG and watch for salt (omit additional salt if it's already included in the spice blend).

Place the fish, chicken, or meat under the grill or on the griddle pan. Cook fish until it is tender and opaque throughout, 7 to 10 minutes, flipping it once. Chicken and meat will take longer, perhaps up to 15 minutes, depending on the thickness. Again, flip it once. The safest way to tell when chicken or meat is done is to check it with a meat thermometer. Chicken is ready when the thermometer registers 75°C; beef is ready at 63°C; and pork and lamb are ready at 71°C. Fish is done once it starts to flake with a fork or when it registers 63°C. Be careful not to overcook your fish, chicken, or meat because it will become dry and tough.

To Sauté:

Sprinkle sea salt, freshly ground black pepper, and any other seasoning you like on your fish, chicken, or meat.

Heat 1 to 2 tablespoons extra-virgin olive oil in a sauté pan over medium-high heat. Place your fish, chicken, or meat in the pan. Turn fish or meat just once while cooking, but turn chicken often to avoid browning it too much on one side. Follow the same cooking times and temperatures as for grilling.

Once it is cooked, season your fish, chicken, or meat with additional sea salt, freshly ground black pepper, up to 1 tablespoon extra-virgin olive oil, and a few squirts of fresh lemon juice. You can also boost the flavor with fresh or dried herbs.

While the recipes in this book are designed to encourage you to cook real, delicious, and inspiring meals, you'll also find that you don't have to follow a recipe or spend hours in the kitchen to follow the program. Just stick to real foods prepared in simple ways and you'll notice that the pounds will come off, the cravings will disappear, and just about every aspect of your health will improve.

PART II

THE RECIPES

My mission is to help people rediscover the joy of eating real food. My personal and professional journey has led me to promote healthy eating. On this journey, I have met remarkable people and discovered amazing organizations. Together we are creating a movement of people who are passionate and ready to make a difference.

As my good friend Steve Sidwell, the founder of Luvo, says, "Food is the problem, but it is also the solution."

I am proud of my association with Luvo and my role as one of their ambassadors. We are working together to put into motion concrete solutions to the problem. Because we believe the solutions should be easy, I have collaborated with John Mitchell, Chief Innovation Officer at Luvo, to create all of the recipes in this book. Our mission is to reinvent "delicious." We want to show that delicious can mean real food with amazing flavor at a reasonable cost. This approach to eating is not about deprivation or starvation or boring, bland diet food. Rather, it is about amazing, delicious, fun, and easy-to-prepare food that makes you feel great.

We hope you will share these meals with your friends and family, and that they become your favorites for generations to come. By buying this book and putting your commitment to healthy eating into action, you too can become a part of the solution.

You now have all of the information you need to embark on your healthy eating journey. One last note: Let this cookbook bring out the inner culinary genius in you. While following recipes is often helpful and inspiring, you don't need recipes in order to eat well. I encourage you to start your own cooking revolution, whether you're following these recipes to a T, editing them to suit your own tastes (a little more garlic, a little less cumin), or abandoning them in favor of your own creations. Have fun, and happy eating!

7

The Basic Plan

BREAKFAST

Strawberry-Almond-Coconut Smoothie

When selecting berries, especially strawberries, choose organic to prevent overloading your system with toxic residue from fertilizers and pesticides. You can likely find frozen organic berries in your local supermarket year-round; they work great in your morning shake.

Serves: 1
Prep Time: 5 minutes

- 1 or 2 large ice cubes
- 2 tablespoons unsalted almond butter
- 175 ml light unsweetened coconut milk
- 120 ml unsweetened almond milk
- 75 g frozen organic strawberries
- 2 teaspoons chia seeds

Combine all of the ingredients in a blender and blend on high until smooth, 1 to 2 minutes. If the smoothie is too thick, add a little water and blend again until it reaches the desired consistency. Drink immediately.

Nutritional analysis per serving: *Calories: 380, Fat: 29 g, Saturated Fat: 8 g, Cholesterol: 0 mg, Fiber: 9 g, Protein: 12 g, Carbohydrates: 13 g, Sodium: 150 mg*

BLUEBERRY-NUT SMOOTHIE

Just 2 Brazil nuts will fulfill your daily need for selenium. Selenium is a powerful antioxidant that helps your immune system stay resilient and also plays a role in a healthy functioning thyroid. Be sure to limit your intake of Brazil nuts to no more than 4 per day, as too much selenium can be bad for you.

Serves: 1
Prep Time: 5 minutes

- 60 g frozen blueberries
- 2 raw Brazil nuts
- 4 raw walnuts
- 115 g non-GMO silken tofu
- 250 ml unsweetened hemp or almond milk
- ½ teaspoon fresh lemon juice
- ¼ teaspoon ground cinnamon
- pinch of sea salt
- 1 or 2 ice cubes

Combine all of the ingredients in a blender and blend on high until smooth, 1 to 2 minutes. If the smoothie is too thick, add a little water and blend again until it reaches the desired consistency. Drink immediately.

Nutritional analysis per serving: *Calories: 252, Fat: 21 g, Saturated Fat: 3 g, Cholesterol: 0 mg, Fiber: 5 g, Protein: 15 g, Carbohydrates: 18 g, Sodium: 248 mg*

Açaı Smoothie

Açai is a type of palm tree native to the Amazon in Brazil. It boasts a load of antioxidants, amino acids, and omega fatty acids. It even contains protein! I love it because its nutrition profile helps put the brakes on the aging process by cooling inflammation and boosting metabolic function as well as eliminating harmful free radicals from our bodies.

Serves: 1
Prep Time: 5 minutes

- 30 g frozen blueberries
- 4 tablespoons frozen açai puree
- 5-mm slice fresh root ginger, peeled
- 3 tablespoons unsweetened hemp protein powder
- 1 tablespoon coconut butter
- 120 ml full-fat unsweetened coconut milk
- 1 or 2 ice cubes (optional)

Combine all of the ingredients in a blender and blend on high speed until smooth, 1 to 2 minutes. If the smoothie is too thick, add a little water and blend again until it reaches the desired consistency. Drink immediately.

Nutritional analysis per serving: *Calories: 295, Fat: 21 g, Saturated Fat: 13 g, Cholesterol: 0 mg, Fiber: 8 g, Protein: 14 g, Carbohydrates: 16 g, Sodium: 250 mg*

CREAMY BERRY SMOOTHIE

I like plant-based protein such as hemp protein powder in my morning smoothie. It is hypoallergenic, which means most people will not have a low-grade inflammatory response to it as some do with soy or dairy. Hemp contains healthy omega fatty acids, protein, antioxidants, fiber, and minerals that support a healthy metabolism and energize your body for a productive morning.

Serves: 1
Prep Time: 5 minutes

- 40 g frozen organic strawberries
- 30 g frozen raspberries
- 115 g non-GMO silken tofu
- 2 tablespoons unsweetened hemp protein powder
- 1 teaspoon fresh lime juice
- 1 or 2 ice cubes (optional)

Combine all of the ingredients in a blender and blend on high speed until smooth, 1 to 2 minutes. If the smoothie is too thick, add a little water and blend again until it reaches the desired consistency. Drink immediately.

Nutritional analysis per serving: *Calories: 257, Fat: 6 g, Saturated Fat: 0 g, Cholesterol: 0 mg, Fiber: 9 g, Protein: 21 g, Carbohydrates: 31 g, Sodium: 13 mg*

ALMOND-BERRY SMOOTHIE

I love this recipe for those mornings when I feel like something refreshing and light yet need real-food energy to carry me through the day. The fiber, protein, and healthy fat in this smoothie keep me going until lunch.

Serves: 1
Prep Time: 5 minutes

- 30 g frozen raspberries
- 30 g frozen blackberries
- 2 tablespoons unsweetened hemp protein powder
- 1 tablespoon flaxseed
- 1 tablespoon unsalted almond butter
- 120 ml unsweetened almond milk
- 1 teaspoon fresh lemon juice
- 1 or 2 ice cubes (optional)

Combine all of the ingredients in a blender and blend on high speed until smooth, 1 to 2 minutes. If the smoothie is too thick, add a little water and blend again until it reaches the desired consistency. Drink immediately.

Nutritional analysis per serving: *Calories: 341, Fat: 19 g, Saturated Fat: 2 g, Cholesterol: 0 mg, Fiber: 11 g, Protein: 21 g, Carbohydrates: 21 g, Sodium: 135 mg*

COCOA-ALMOND SMOOTHIE

When selecting cocoa products, try to find raw cacao powder in your local supermarket or order online. Raw cacao is less processed than cocoa and yields higher amounts of minerals, vitamins, healthy fats, and fiber.

Serves: 1
Prep Time: 5 minutes

- 2 or 3 large ice cubes
- 300 ml unsweetened almond milk
- 2 tablespoons unsalted almond butter
- 1 tablespoon chia seeds
- 2 teaspoons unsweetened cocoa powder
- 1 tablespoon coconut oil

Combine all of the ingredients in a blender and blend on high speed until smooth, 1 to 2 minutes. If the smoothie is too thick, add a little water and blend again until it reaches the desired consistency. Drink immediately.

Nutritional analysis per serving: *Calories: 430, Fat: 39 g, Saturated Fat: 14 g, Cholesterol: 0 mg, Fiber: 9 g, Protein: 10 g, Carbohydrates: 14 g, Sodium: 300 mg*

CRUSTLESS ASPARAGUS QUICHE

I love a good quiche to start off my weekend.

Serves: 4
Prep Time: 15 minutes
Cook Time: 20 minutes

- 1¾ teaspoons sea salt
- 8 asparagus spears, trimmed
- 10 large omega-3 eggs
- 2 shallots, finely chopped
- 4 tablespoons coarsely chopped fresh dill
- 2 teaspoons grapeseed oil
- 1 avocado, stoned, peeled, and sliced, for garnish

Preheat the oven to 220°C/Gas 7.

Bring a 3-liter saucepan of water to the boil over high heat. Add 1 teaspoon of the sea salt. Add the asparagus to the boiling water and cook until bright green and crisp-tender, 1 to 2 minutes. Transfer the asparagus to a colander and rinse with cold water until cool. Dry the asparagus thoroughly with kitchen paper. Set aside.

In a large bowl, whisk together the eggs, shallots, dill, and remaining ¾ teaspoon salt.

Place a 24 cm by 5-cm-deep nonstick quiche tin with a removable bottom on a rimmed baking sheet. Wrap the bottom of the tin tightly with aluminium foil. Using a pastry brush, lightly grease the tin with the grapeseed oil. Spread the asparagus evenly in the bottom of the tin. Pour the egg mixture over the asparagus.

Place the baking sheet in the center of the oven and bake until the quiche is puffed and golden and a cocktail stick inserted in the center comes out clean, 15 to 17 minutes. Cool for 10 minutes before removing from the tin. Serve, garnished with sliced avocado.

Nutritional analysis per serving: *Calories: 210, Fat: 14 g, Saturated Fat: 3.5 g, Cholesterol: 450 mg, Fiber: 1 g, Protein: 16 g, Carbohydrates: 6 g, Sodium: 421 mg*

VEGETABLE HASH WITH FRIED EGGS

If you don't have time to make this in the morning, make the hash a few days ahead, store it in the refrigerator, and then reheat it in a sauté pan or cast-iron frying pan.

Serves: 4
Prep Time: 10 minutes
Cook Time: 30 minutes

- 2 tablespoons extra-virgin olive oil
- 1 medium onion, diced
- 1 medium white or green cabbage, diced
- 1 organic red pepper, seeded and diced
- 1 organic green pepper, seeded and diced
- 8 asparagus spears, trimmed and cut into 5-mm pieces
- 2 spring onions, thinly sliced
- ½ teaspoon dried oregano
- ½ teaspoon dried thyme
- ½ teaspoon dried sage
- ¼ teaspoon sea salt
- pinch of freshly ground black pepper
- 8 large omega-3 eggs
- ½ ripe avocado, stoned, peeled, and sliced, for garnish
- chopped fresh basil or parsley, for garnish

Preheat the oven to 200°C/Gas 6.

Heat the oil in a large oven-proof sauté pan or cast-iron frying pan over medium heat for 30 seconds. Add the onion and sauté, stirring occasionally, until lightly caramelized and golden, 5 to 7 minutes.

Add the cabbage and sauté until soft and golden, 7 to 8 minutes. Add the peppers and sauté until they begin to caramelize, about 5 minutes. Add the asparagus and spring onions and cook for an additional 1 to 2 minutes, or just until the asparagus turns bright green.

Season the vegetables with the dried herbs, salt, and black pepper.

Make four small wells in the surface of the hash, each about the size of a lemon, and carefully break two eggs into each well.

Place the pan in the oven and bake until the eggs are set, 5 to 7 minutes. (Alternatively, you can poach or fry the eggs, then serve them on individual plates of hash.)

Garnish each egg with avocado and fresh herbs and serve.

Nutritional analysis per serving: Calories: 280, Fat: 19 g, Saturated Fat: 4 g, Cholesterol: 360 mg, Fiber: 5 g, Protein: 15 g, Carbohydrates: 14 g, Sodium: 290 mg

Southwestern Vegetable Frittata

Frittatas are a great way to use up leftovers, and you can feel free to add other cooked vegetables than the ones mentioned here. Try chopped cooked broccoli, grilled courgettes and peppers, or sautéed spinach.

Serves: 4
Prep Time: 10 minutes
Cook Time: 35 minutes

- 8 large omega-3 eggs
- ½ teaspoon mild chili powder
- 1 tablespoon finely chopped fresh chives and/or basil
- sea salt and freshly ground black pepper
- 1 tablespoon extra-virgin olive oil
- ¼ red onion, thinly sliced
- ½ small head white cabbage, finely diced
- 1 garlic clove, finely chopped
- 150 g finely shredded kale leaves or other leafy greens
- 16 roasted cherry tomatoes (see Note)
- 1 ripe avocado, stoned, peeled, and diced, for garnish
- salsa, for garnish (optional)

Preheat the oven to 190°C/Gas 5.

In a bowl, whisk together the eggs, chili powder, herbs, ½ teaspoon salt, and a pinch of black pepper.

Heat the olive oil in a 20-cm nonstick oven-proof frying pan over medium heat until shimmering.

Add the red onion to the pan and sauté for 1 minute, then add the cabbage. Sauté the cabbage until it's wilted and beginning to brown, about 5 minutes. Add the garlic and kale to the pan and cook until the kale is wilted and very soft, about 5 minutes more. Season the vegetables with a pinch of salt.

Pour the egg mixture over the vegetables and scatter the roasted tomatoes over the eggs. Place the pan in the oven and bake until the eggs are fully set but the center is just barely soft, 18 to 22 minutes. Remove the frittata from the oven and allow it to rest for 5 minutes. Cut into 4 wedges and serve, garnished with avocado and salsa, if desired.

Note: To make the roasted cherry tomatoes, preheat the oven to 200°C/ Gas 6. Toss 450 g cherry tomatoes with 1 tablespoon of extra-virgin olive oil and a pinch of salt, and spread them out on a rimmed baking sheet. Roast the tomatoes until they are shriveled and starting to brown, about 30 minutes. Let them cool for 5 minutes, then transfer them to an airtight container and store in the refrigerator for up to 5 days. They can be added to salads, stews, and sauces, or mashed up with basil as a delicious topping for grilled meats and fish.

Nutritional analysis per serving (does not include salsa): *Calories: 240, Fat: 16 g, Saturated Fat: 3.5 g, Cholesterol: 360 mg, Fiber: 4 g, Protein: 15 g, Carbohydrates: 11 g, Sodium: 450 mg*

ASPARAGUS AND MUSHROOM FRITTATA WITH TOMATO COULIS

Coulis is a French culinary term to describe a thick puree. Here, the tomato coulis balances the pungent flavor of the onion and the earthiness of the mushrooms. This frittata will make you feel as if you just enjoyed brunch at your local brasserie without even leaving home!

Serves: 4
Prep Time: 20 minutes
Cook Time: 20 minutes

- 2 tomatoes, cored and quartered
- 2 oil-packed sun-dried tomatoes
- 1 small garlic clove
- 1 teaspoon sea salt
- ½ teaspoon freshly ground black pepper
- 3 tablespoons extra-virgin olive oil
- 1 large red onion, finely chopped
- 450 g asparagus, trimmed and cut on the bias into 2.5-cm pieces
- 225 g chestnut mushrooms, trimmed and thinly sliced
- 6 large omega-3 eggs

To make the tomato coulis, combine the fresh tomatoes, sun-dried tomatoes, garlic, and ¼ teaspoon each salt and black pepper in a blender or food processor. Puree until smooth. Set aside.

Heat 2 tablespoons of the oil in a 23-cm nonstick frying pan over medium heat until shimmering. Add the onion, sprinkle with ¼ teaspoon salt, and cook, stirring occasionally, until just translucent, about 7 minutes.

Add the asparagus and mushrooms, sprinkle with another ¼ teaspoon salt, and cook, stirring occasionally, until the asparagus is crisp-tender and the juices released by the mushrooms evaporate, about 6 minutes.

Meanwhile, in a bowl, whisk the eggs with the remaining ¼ teaspoon each salt and black pepper. Add the asparagus mixture to the eggs and stir gently.

Heat the remaining 1 tablespoon oil in the same pan over medium heat until shimmering. Pour the egg mixture into the pan and fold gently, pull-ing the cooked edges in to evenly cook the eggs.

When the egg mixture starts to set, spread it out in an even layer, cover, and cook until fully set, about 3 minutes. Uncover and loosen the frittata before inverting or sliding onto a serving plate. Cut into wedges and serve with the tomato coulis spooned over the top.

Nutritional analysis per serving: *Calories: 260, Fat: 18 g, Saturated Fat: 3.5 g, Cholesterol: 270 mg, Fiber: 4 g, Protein: 14 g, Carbohydrates: 15 g, Sodium: 523 mg*

Wild Mushroom and Leek Frittata

While it makes a great breakfast, a frittata can also be served with a green salad for lunch or even a light dinner. Make sure your wild mushrooms come from a reputable source—a farmers' market is best. Don't be intimidated by using leeks; they're simple to clean and delicious.

Serves: 4
Prep Time: 15 minutes
Cook Time: 35 minutes

- 4 tablespoons plus 1 teaspoon grapeseed oil
- 1 large leek, cut into 1-cm-thick slices
- 175 g wild mushrooms, stalks removed and cut into 5-mm-thick slices
- 2 teaspoons fresh thyme
- ¾ teaspoon sea salt
- pinch of cayenne pepper, or to taste
- 8 large omega-3 eggs, beaten
- ½ small bunch chives, thinly sliced, for garnish

Preheat the oven to 220°C/Gas 7.

Heat 1 teaspoon of the oil in a large oven-proof frying pan over medium–low heat until shimmering. Add the leek and cook until tender, 6 to 8 minutes. Transfer the leek to a bowl and set aside.

Add 2 tablespoons of the oil to the pan and raise the temperature to medium-high. When the pan is hot, add half of the mushrooms; cook, stirring occasionally, until they are deep golden-brown, 3 to 4 minutes. If the bottom of the pan begins to get dark, add 4 tablespoons water and use a flexible rubber spatula to loosen the dark bits. Add the cooked mushrooms to the reserved leeks.

Return the pan to the heat. Repeat the process with the remaining 2 tablespoons oil and the remaining mushrooms. Once the second batch of mushrooms is cooked, return the leek and mushroom mixture to the pan.

Add the thyme, salt, and cayenne pepper to the pan and stir to combine.

Remove the pan from the heat, add the eggs, and quickly stir to combine the ingredients.

Place the pan in the oven on the center shelf. Cook until golden brown, puffed, and set (a cocktail stick inserted in the center should come out clean), 13 to 15 minutes. Allow to cool for 5 minutes before running a flexible rubber spatula around the edges and then carefully underneath the frittata to loosen it from the bottom of the pan. Slide the frittata onto a plate, cut into wedges, and serve garnished with about 1 tablespoon of chives per wedge.

Note: The frittata can be served cold. Allow it to come to room temperature before covering and chilling.

Nutritional analysis per serving: *Calories: 300, Fat: 24 g, Saturated Fat: 4 g, Cholesterol: 360 mg, Fiber: 2 g, Protein: 13 g, Carbohydrates: 8 g, Sodium: 550 mg*

TURKEY SAUSAGE PATTIES

Enjoy a serving of sausage patties with a fried egg or scrambled eggs mixed with chopped cooked asparagus and some fresh berries alongside.

Serves: 4
Prep Time: 10 minutes
Cook Time: 10 minutes

- 450 g lean minced turkey
- 2½ teaspoons fennel seeds
- 1 teaspoon dried oregano
- 1 teaspoon dried thyme
- 1 teaspoon sweet paprika
- ½ teaspoon crushed chili flakes
- ½ teaspoon sea salt
- ¼ teaspoon freshly ground black pepper
- 1 tablespoon avocado or grapeseed oil
- 200 g fresh berries

In a bowl, combine the minced turkey and all of the spices, salt, and black pepper. Use your hands to combine the mixture, making sure the spices are well mixed into the minced turkey. Form the meat into 8 equal-size patties.

Heat the oil in a large nonstick frying pan over medium–high heat until shimmering. Sauté the patties until brown on both sides and cooked through, 8 to 10 minutes, using a heat-proof spatula to press down and flatten the patties a few times as they cook. Check to make sure the turkey is fully cooked by cutting into the center of one patty (no pink should remain) or checking that the internal temperature measures 75°C.

Serve 2 patties with 50 g berries.

Nutritional analysis per serving: *Calories: 252, Fat: 13 g, Saturated Fat: 3 g, Cholesterol: 84 mg, Fiber: 3 g, Protein: 22 g, Carbohydrates: 12 g, Sodium: 321 mg*

Poached Eggs over Spinach with Braised Artichoke Bottoms

Poaching is a fast and healthy way to cook eggs. Because the yolk is not exposed to high heat for too long, the essential fats as well as important fat-soluble vitamins and antioxidants—like lutein—do not break down.

Serves: 4
Prep Time: 15 minutes
Cook Time: 15 minutes

- 2 teaspoons extra-virgin olive oil
- 500 g organic spinach
- sea salt
- 2 (400-g) cans artichoke bottoms, rinsed and drained
- 8 large omega-3 eggs, plus 1 yolk
- 120 ml Mayonnaise (page 299) or Vegenaise
- 1 teaspoon Dijon mustard
- grated zest and juice of 1 lemon
- 1 garlic clove, halved
- $\frac{1}{8}$ teaspoon cayenne pepper
- 2 teaspoons distilled vinegar or additional fresh lemon juice, for poaching
- paprika, for garnish

Preheat the grill. Line a baking sheet with aluminium foil and brush the foil with 1 teaspoon of the oil. Set aside.

In a large nonstick frying pan, heat the remaining 1 teaspoon oil over medium-high heat until shimmering. Add the spinach and toss until slightly wilted. Season with a pinch of salt. Cover and cook for 1 minute. Transfer to a colander and press out any excess liquid from the spinach.

Slice off the underside of each artichoke bottom so that they sit flat. Place the artichoke bottoms on the prepared baking sheet and grill until warm and slightly golden, about 3 minutes. Set aside.

While the artichokes cook, combine the egg yolk, mayonnaise, mustard, lemon zest and juice, garlic, cayenne, ½ teaspoon salt, and 2 tablespoons cold water in a food processor and pulse until the mixture reaches a creamy, sauce-like consistency.

Bring 1 liter of water to a simmer in a medium saucepan over medium-high heat. Add the vinegar to the simmering water. Crack 1 egg into a small bowl and gently tip the egg into the water. Quickly repeat with 3 more eggs, being careful not to let the eggs touch. Cook until the whites are set and the yolks are runny, 2 to 3 minutes. With a slotted spoon, transfer the eggs to a plate lined with kitchen paper to drain. Repeat with the remaining 4 eggs.

Place two artichoke bottoms on each plate. Top each with cooked spinach and an egg, then a spoonful of sauce. Garnish with a sprinkle of paprika and serve.

Nutritional analysis per serving: *Calories: 342, Fat: 28 g, Saturated Fat: 6 g, Cholesterol: 432 mg, Fiber: 13 g, Protein: 19 g, Carbohydrates: 20 g, Sodium: 580 mg*

Spinach-Mushroom-Asparagus Strata

Concerned about eggs raising your cholesterol? Don't be! This nutrition myth constantly surprises my patients. It turns out that cholesterol from food is not the culprit—sugar is! By enjoying seven to eight omega-3 eggs per week, you increase your antioxidant intake and receive healthy amounts of fat, protein, and nutrition—all of which help lower your cholesterol, not raise it.

Serves: 4
Prep Time: 15 minutes
Cook Time: 1 hour

- 3 teaspoons coconut oil
- 900 g chestnut mushrooms, trimmed and sliced
- 300 g organic baby spinach
- 2 garlic cloves, finely chopped
- 1½ tablespoons pine nuts
- 450 g asparagus, trimmed
- 8 large omega-3 eggs
- 75 ml unsweetened almond milk
- 2 tablespoons nutritional yeast, plus more for optional garnish
- 1 spring onion, finely chopped
- 1 jalapeño chili, seeded and finely chopped (optional)
- ¼ teaspoon sea salt
- ¼ teaspoon freshly ground black pepper

Preheat the oven to 180°C/Gas 4. Lightly coat a 20-cm square baking dish with 1 teaspoon of the coconut oil; set aside.

Warm 1 teaspoon of the coconut oil in a large nonstick sauté pan over medium-high heat until shimmering. Add the mushrooms and sauté until they have released their liquid and that liquid has evaporated, 8 to 10 minutes. Transfer the mushrooms to a bowl and set aside.

In the same pan, warm the remaining 1 teaspoon coconut oil over medium heat until shimmering. Add half of the spinach, stirring constantly until wilted, 2 to 3 minutes. Add the remaining spinach, stirring again and cooking until wilted, another 2 minutes. Stir in the garlic and pine nuts; cook for 30 seconds. Remove the pan from the heat and set aside.

Transfer half of the mushrooms to the bottom of the prepared baking dish. Top with half of the spinach. Layer half of the asparagus spears on top of the spinach. Repeat with the remaining mushrooms, spinach, and asparagus.

In a small bowl, whisk together the eggs and almond milk. Add the nutritional yeast, spring onion, jalapeño (if using), salt, and black pepper, whisking to combine. Pour the egg mixture evenly into the baking dish.

Bake until the center is firm to the touch, 40 to 50 minutes. A little of the moisture from the vegetables will rise to the top; blot with kitchen paper, if desired.

Cut the strata into 4 squares and serve, garnished with additional nutritional yeast, if desired.

Nutritional analysis per serving: *Calories: 293, Fat: 15 g, Saturated Fat: 5 g, Cholesterol: 350 mg, Fiber: 9 g, Protein: 25 g, Carbohydrates: 25 g, Sodium: 318 mg*

Spicy Scrambled Tofu
with Courgettes and Coriander

I encourage my community to avoid all genetically modified soy because of the hazardous health effects it carries.

Serves: 4
Prep Time: 10 minutes
Cook Time: 20 minutes

- 5 tablespoons extra-virgin olive oil
- 3 small courgettes, cut into 2.5-cm cubes
- 1 small onion, chopped
- 3 garlic cloves, finely chopped
- 1 green bird's eye chili, seeded and finely chopped
- 1 teaspoon grated fresh root ginger
- ¼ teaspoon crushed chili flakes
- 450 g organic spinach, stalks removed
- 400 g non-GMO extra-firm tofu, drained and crumbled
- ½ teaspoon sea salt
- 4 tablespoons roughly chopped fresh coriander

Heat 3 tablespoons of the oil in a 30-cm frying pan over high heat until shimmering. Add the courgettes and cook until browned on all sides and tender, 6 to 8 minutes. Transfer to a large bowl.

Add the onion, garlic, chili, ginger, and chili flakes to the pan and cook until the onion is translucent, 3 to 5 minutes. Add to the bowl.

Add the spinach to the pan and cook, stirring often, until just wilted, 2 to 3 minutes. Add the spinach to the courgette and onion mixture.

Heat the remaining 2 tablespoons oil in the pan over medium heat until shimmering. Add the tofu and cook, stirring, until heated through, 3 to 5 minutes. Add the tofu to the courgette mixture. Season with the salt, stir in the chopped coriander, and serve.

Nutritional analysis per serving: *Calories: 320, Fat: 23 g, Saturated Fat: 3.5 g, Cholesterol: 0 mg, Fiber: 8 g, Protein: 14 g, Carbohydrates: 20 g, Sodium: 340 mg*

LUNCH

Dr. Hyman's Super Salad Bar

Why go to a salad bar when you can create your own at home? As always, preparation is the key to a successful detox. To get our kitchens and ourselves prepared to enjoy a delicious salad from home, be sure to take a little time to set up your own salad bar fixings. Here's what to do:

- Wash and cut veggies into convenient salad-size bits and store them in sealed glass containers all in one location in your refrigerator. Cut enough for 2 to 3 days and repeat throughout the 10 days as needed for freshness. Add different veggies at least twice a week for variety.
- Make a salad for lunch the night before so you can grab-and-go on your way out the door. Store dressing in a separate container.
- Store items not requiring refrigeration in small glass jars, preferably on a single shelf so they're easy to find. Toasted and raw nuts and seeds stay fresh for weeks at room temperature when sealed in glass jars.
- Ready, set, prep: Pick a variety of items from the list below and add them to your shopping list each week. Start by choosing your greens. Consider mixing various types of greens—I like having some romaine with rocket to balance out texture. (Skip iceberg lettuce; it is hardly green and has almost no nutrients.) Then choose your veggies, protein, healthy fats, and dressing. Select different options each day to keep your palate happy.

GREENS (60 G PER SALAD)

- Rocket
- Spinach (organic when possible)
- Romaine

- Watercress
- Kale
- Mixed baby leaves

VEGETABLES (125 TO 250 G PER SALAD EXCEPT AS NOTED)

- Cucumbers (organic when possible)
- Peppers: red, green, yellow (organic when possible)
- Sprouts: sunflower, pea shoots, clover, etc.
- Tomatoes: baby plum, cherry (organic when possible)
- Carrots
- Broccoli
- Cauliflower
- Cabbage: red, Chinese leaves, etc.
- Mushrooms
- Sugarsnap peas (organic when possible)
- Steamed asparagus
- Artichoke hearts (packed in water in glass jars)
- Hearts of palm (packed in water in glass jars)
- Courgettes
- Roasted aubergines
- Roasted or steamed beetroot (40 to 75 g)
- Red onions (40 to 75 g)
- Spring onions (40 to 75 g)
- Herbs: parsley, basil, oregano, dill, coriander, mint, oregano, etc. (4 tablespoons fresh and/or 1 teaspoon dried)

PROTEIN (100 TO 175 G)

- Canned fish (in water): salmon, sardines, herring, etc. (Skip tuna; it has too much mercury.)
- Chicken (baked or roasted)
- Turkey (baked or roasted)
- Tofu
- Tempeh

- Hard–boiled eggs (2)
- Cooked prawns or other seafood

HEALTHY FATS (CHOOSE ONE)

- Avocado (¼ to ½)
- Nuts, raw: almonds, cashews, walnuts, hazelnuts, pecans, etc. (4 tablespoons)
- Seeds, raw: flax, chia, hemp, sunflower, pumpkin, sesame, etc. (4 tablespoons)
- Kalamata olives (4 tablespoons)

DRESSING (1 TO 2 TABLESPOONS PER SALAD)

Start by mixing oil (extra–virgin olive oil, flaxseed oil, walnut oil, or avocado oil) and fresh lemon or lime juice or vinegar (or a combination) at a ratio of two–thirds oil to one–third lemon or vinegar. Whisk in any of these to taste:

- Dijon mustard
- Seasonings, including salt and black pepper; fresh or dried herbs such as basil, oregano, or rosemary; and finely chopped garlic or onion. For creamy dressing, add avocado or tahini (sesame paste).

Blanched Asparagus with Soft-Boiled Eggs

I love anchovies. Contrary to popular belief they don't taste "fishy" but rather slightly savory and salty. A little anchovy packs a lot of flavor, so you don't need many to get a burst of flavor from these heart–healthy fish.

Serves: 4
Prep Time: 5 minutes
Cook Time: 10 minutes

- 8 large omega-3 eggs
- sea salt
- 900 g asparagus, trimmed
- 4 tablespoons halved Niçoise olives
- 4 oil-packed anchovy fillets, coarsely chopped
- 2 tablespoons extra-virgin olive oil
- 4 tablespoons roughly chopped fresh basil
- ¼ teaspoon freshly ground black pepper

Put the eggs in a large saucepan and add enough cold water to cover by 2.5 cm. Bring the water to the boil over medium heat; remove from the heat and cover. Let stand for 2 minutes (see Note). Use a slotted spoon to transfer the eggs to a bowl; reserve the hot water in the pan. Cover the eggs with cold water and set aside.

Return the water in the pan to the boil over medium-high heat and add 2 teaspoons salt. Add the asparagus and cook until bright green and almost crisp-tender, about 4 minutes. Drain and arrange in a single layer on four serving plates. Scatter the olives and anchovies evenly over the asparagus.

Lightly crack 2 eggs over each bed of asparagus and scoop them out, letting the yolks run over the asparagus. Sprinkle the eggs with a pinch of salt. Drizzle the olive oil over each serving and scatter the basil leaves on top. Sprinkle with the black pepper and serve.

Nutritional analysis per serving: *Calories: 281, Fat: 19 g, Saturated Fat: 4 g, Cholesterol: 363 mg, Fiber: 5 g, Protein: 18 g, Carbohydrates: 12 g, Sodium: 507 mg*

CHERRY TOMATO AND TOFU SALAD

This salad gets better the longer it sits, as the tofu soaks up the dressing and tomato juices. It is lovely served on a bed of peppery rocket leaves.

Serves: 4
Prep Time: 10 minutes, plus resting time

- 2 teaspoons gluten-free, low-sodium tamari
- 2 teaspoons toasted sesame oil
- 1 teaspoon balsamic vinegar
- 2 tablespoons extra-virgin olive oil
- 1.3 kg cherry tomatoes, halved
- 3 tablespoons raw pumpkin seeds
- 2 teaspoons sesame seeds
- 400 g non-GMO extra-firm tofu, drained and cut into 2.5-cm cubes
- ¼ teaspoon sea salt
- ¼ teaspoon freshly ground black pepper
- 1 avocado, stoned, peeled, and chopped
- 4 tablespoons thinly sliced fresh mint

In a large bowl, combine the tamari, sesame oil, and balsamic vinegar. Whisk in the olive oil.

Add the tomatoes to the bowl, stirring to combine with the dressing. Stir in the pumpkin and sesame seeds.

Add the tofu cubes and season with the salt and black pepper. Gently toss. Let sit for 30 minutes at room temperature, so the tofu absorbs the dressing. (The salad can also sit in the refrigerator, covered, for up to 1 day prior to serving.)

Top with the chopped avocado and mint and serve.

Nutritional analysis per serving: *Calories: 350, Fat: 26 g, Saturated Fat: 3.5 g, Cholesterol: 0 mg, Fiber: 7 g, Protein: 15 g, Carbohydrates: 17 g, Sodium: 310 mg*

THAI TOFU AND AVOCADO SALAD
WITH CHILI-LIME DRESSING

Look for organic, extra-firm tofu, which has a pleasing chewy texture and will also soak up the dressing really well.

Serves: 4
Prep Time: 15 minutes, plus resting time

- 400 g non-GMO extra-firm tofu, drained and cut into 1-cm cubes
- ¼ teaspoon ground turmeric
- 2 tablespoons extra-virgin olive oil
- 1 tablespoon fresh lime juice
- 1 tablespoon Thai fish sauce
- Pinch chili flakes
- 150 g shredded Chinese leaves or green cabbage
- ½ large cucumber, thinly sliced
- 4 plum tomatoes, cut into eighths
- ½ small red onion or 1 shallot, finely sliced
- 20 g roughly chopped mixed fresh herbs (such as coriander, mint, and/or basil)
- 2 tablespoons flaked or sliced almonds
- ½ avocado, stoned, peeled, and diced

Place the tofu in a large salad bowl and sprinkle with the turmeric. Toss well to combine. Set aside.

In a small bowl, whisk together the olive oil, lime juice, fish sauce, and chili flakes. Pour half of the dressing over the tofu and set aside for 30 minutes to allow it to marinate while you cut up the vegetables. Set aside the remaining dressing.

Add the Chinese leaves, cucumber, tomatoes, and onion to the tofu. Add the remaining dressing to the salad and toss well to combine. Garnish with the herbs, almonds, and avocado and serve.

Nutritional analysis per serving: *Calories: 240, Fat: 17 g, Saturated Fat: 3 g, Cholesterol: 0 mg, Fiber: 5 g, Protein: 13 g, Carbohydrates: 11 g, Sodium: 370 mg*

BRUSSELS SPROUTS AND BROCCOLI SLAW WITH SEARED SCALLOPS

Gram for gram, broccoli stems have the same nutrition as the florets. When you eat real food you can be sure that for the most part, the whole food can be consumed and will provide nutrition that our bodies can use to flourish.

Serves: 4
Prep Time: 15 minutes
Cook Time: 10 minutes

- 450 g Brussels sprouts, trimmed
- 800 g broccoli, stems peeled, florets cut into bite-size pieces
- 4 tablespoons finely sliced fresh basil
- 4 tablespoons fresh lemon juice
- 4 tablespoons balsamic vinegar
- 3 tablespoons extra-virgin olive oil
- sea salt and freshly ground black pepper
- 16 large scallops, patted dry, tough muscles discarded

Fit the shredding blade into a food processor. Process the Brussels sprouts and broccoli stems until finely shredded. Transfer to a large bowl. Add the basil, lemon juice, 2 tablespoons of the vinegar, 1 tablespoon of the oil, ¼ teaspoon salt, and a pinch of black pepper. Toss until mixed well. Set the slaw aside.

Heat 1 tablespoon of the oil in a large frying pan over high heat until shimmering. Season the scallops with ¼ teaspoon salt and ½ teaspoon black pepper. Add the scallops to the pan in a single layer without crowding; work in batches, if necessary. Cook until dark brown on the bottom, 1 to 2 minutes, and then flip and brown the other side, 1 to 2 minutes more. Transfer to a plate.

Add the remaining 1 tablespoon oil to the pan and heat until shimmering. Add the broccoli florets in an even layer. Sprinkle with a pinch each of salt and black pepper. Add 2 tablespoons of water, cover, and cook until the broccoli is crisp-tender and browned on the bottom, about 3 minutes. Transfer to the slaw.

Add the remaining 2 tablespoons vinegar to the pan and simmer until slightly thickened, about 30 seconds. To serve, divide the slaw among four serving plates, top with 4 scallops per plate, and drizzle with the reduced balsamic.

Nutritional analysis per serving: *Calories: 325, Fat: 13 g, Saturated Fat: 2 g, Cholesterol: 37 mg, Fiber: 10 g, Protein: 29 g, Carbohydrates: 30 g, Sodium: 570 mg*

FENNEL SALAD WITH ROAST COD FILLETS

Cod is one of my favorite fish because it is mild yet firm and flaky, so it can take on the flavors of your meal, making for a great canvas. Enjoy the health benefits of cod in this easy-to-make, delicious salad.

Serves: 4
Prep Time: 10 minutes
Cook Time: 30 minutes

- 2 fennel bulbs, trimmed and finely sliced
- 4 tablespoons plus 1 teaspoon grapeseed oil
- sea salt and freshly ground black pepper
- 2 peppers (red and/or yellow), seeded and cut into strips
- 1 large onion, cut into 8 wedges
- 2 tablespoons sweet paprika
- 2 (350-g) wild-caught cod fillets
- 1 tablespoons extra-virgin olive oil
- 1 tablespoon balsamic vinegar
- 1 teaspoon Dijon mustard
- 2 small heads round lettuce, roughly torn

Preheat the oven to 230°C/Gas 8. Line two rimmed baking sheets with aluminium foil.

In a medium bowl, toss the fennel with 2 tablespoons of the grapeseed oil, ½ teaspoon salt, and a pinch of black pepper. Spread evenly on one of the lined baking sheets.

Put the peppers and onion in the same bowl and toss with another 2 tablespoons grapeseed oil, ½ teaspoon salt, and a pinch of black pepper. Spread evenly on the other lined baking sheet.

Roast the fennel on the bottom shelf of the oven and the peppers and onion on the middle rack until the fennel has browned on the bottom, 12 to 15 minutes. Give all of the vegetables a toss to prevent burning and continue to cook until they are all golden brown, another 5 to 7 minutes. Remove from the oven, transfer to a large bowl, and set aside.

In a small bowl, whisk the paprika into 4 tablespoons cold water.

Remove the foil and brush one of the baking sheets with the remaining 1 teaspoon grapeseed oil and place the cod fillets on the sheet. Baste with about half of the paprika mixture. Roast until the cod is opaque through-out, basting again with the remaining paprika mixture halfway through. Fish typically takes about 12 minutes to cook per 2.5 cm of thickness.

While the fish is baking, whisk together the olive oil, vinegar, mustard, and a pinch of salt in a small bowl. Add to the bowl of roasted vegetables and toss to coat.

Divide the lettuce among four serving plates and top with the roasted vegetables.

When the fish is done, use a fork to gently flake the fillets into bite-size pieces. Arrange the cod on top of the fennel salad and serve.

Nutritional analysis per serving: *Calories: 410, Fat: 21 g, Saturated Fat: 2.5 g, Cholesterol: 75 mg, Fiber: 9 g, Protein: 30 g, Carbohydrates: 23 g, Sodium: 490 mg*

GREEK SALAD WITH MACKEREL

This salad is made for your 10-Day Detox Diet because it contains ingredients that are powerful detoxification agents. Onion, oregano, lemon, mackerel, olive oil, and vegetables contain potent nutrients to boost your metabolism.

Serves: 4
Prep Time: 15 minutes
Cook Time: 5 minutes

- 1 tablespoon finely chopped fresh oregano
- 4 tablespoons extra-virgin olive oil
- 4 (175-g) boneless wild mackerel fillets
- sea salt and freshly ground black pepper
- 2 large heads romaine lettuce, chopped
- 150 g heirloom tomatoes, diced
- 1 cucumber, diced
- 1 large yellow pepper, seeded and very thinly sliced
- ¼ red onion, very thinly sliced
- 75 g pitted Kalamata olives
- 4 tablespoons fresh lemon juice

Heat a well-seasoned griddle pan over medium heat.

In a large bowl, whisk the chopped oregano into the oil.

Rub 1 tablespoon of the oregano-oil mixture all over the mackerel fillets. Season the fillets with ½ teaspoon salt and ¼ teaspoon black pepper. Place the fillets on the hot griddle pan and grill until the flesh is just opaque throughout, about 5 minutes, turning once during grilling. Transfer to a chopping board and cut each fillet into thirds.

Add the lettuce, tomatoes, cucumber, pepper, onion, and olives to the remaining oregano-oil mixture. Sprinkle with a pinch each of salt and black pepper. Toss until well coated. Add the lemon juice and toss again. Divide the salad among four serving plates, top with the grilled mackerel, and serve.

Nutritional analysis per serving: *Calories: 460, Fat: 29 g, Saturated Fat: 5 g, Cholesterol: 130 mg, Fiber: 4 g, Protein: 36 g, Carbohydrates: 15 g, Sodium: 550 mg*

Spring Greens with Grilled Salmon

I love any recipe that has lemon or lime juice for the flavor-enhancing effects it has on the entire meal, so the fact that this recipe has both makes it a favorite in my home. If you prefer, feel free to substitute any hearty greens for the spring greens, such as kale, Swiss chard or mustard greens.

Serves: 4
Prep Time: 25 minutes
Cook Time: 10 minutes

- juice of 1 lemon, plus grated zest of ½ lemon
- juice of 2 limes, plus grated zest of 1 lime
- 2½ tablespoons extra-virgin olive oil
- sea salt and freshly ground black pepper
- 1 to 2 large bunches mustard greens, roughly torn
- 25 g parsley leaves
- ¼ small red onion, thinly sliced
- coconut oil, for coating grill
- 1 tablespoon Dijon mustard
- 4 (115- to 175-g) boneless, skin-on wild salmon fillets

In a small bowl, whisk together the citrus juices and zests.

In a separate small bowl prepare the dressing by whisking together 2 tablespoons of the citrus mixture, the olive oil, ¼ teaspoon salt, and a pinch of black pepper.

Place the greens in a large bowl, add the dressing, and gently massage the greens with your hands until the salad has wilted to almost half its original size, 2 to 3 minutes. Stir in the parsley and onion and set aside.

Prepare the grill for medium to medium-high heat, or heat a well-seasoned griddle pan over medium-high heat. Lightly coat the grill or griddle pan with coconut oil to prevent sticking.

In a small bowl, whisk together the mustard, remaining citrus mixture, and ¼ teaspoon each salt and black pepper. Using a spoon or a brush, spread the mustard mixture over the flesh side of the salmon fillets. Place the salmon fillets, skin-side up, on the grill or griddle pan. Cook to the desired doneness, 4 to 5 minutes per side.

Divide the salad among four serving plates, place a salmon fillet on each plate, and serve.

Nutritional analysis per serving: *Calories: 290, Fat: 16 g, Saturated Fat: 2 g, Cholesterol: 60 mg, Fiber: 6 g, Protein: 27 g, Carbohydrates: 11 g, Sodium: 480 mg*

Prawn and Mangetout Salad

This salad celebrates one of my favorite low-glycemic vegetables—jicama. Jicama (pronounced hee-ka-ma) is a nutrition powerhouse of fiber, potassium, vitamin C, and other antioxidants. It also contains the fiber inulin, which is a prebiotic that helps nourish our intestinal tract, allowing for healthy gut flora to flourish. A healthy microbiome is important for immunity, disease prevention, mood, and even keeping cravings away. Jicama can be found in speciality Mexican shops and in the specialist food sections of some supermarkets. Water chestnuts or daikon radish (mooli) could be used as a substitute.

Serves: 4
Prep Time: 30 minutes, plus marinating time
Cook Time: 5 minutes

- ½ teaspoon sea salt
- 450 g mangetout, trimmed and cut into strips
- 450 g raw prawns, peeled and deveined
- 2 teaspoons grated fresh lime zest
- 250 ml fresh lime juice (from 8 to 10 limes)
- 4 tablespoons extra-virgin olive oil
- 1 or 2 red chilies (such as Anaheim or Fresno), seeded and finely chopped
- 1 small shallot, thinly sliced
- 60 g jicama, chopped
- 5 tablespoons chopped fresh coriander

Bring a 5-liter saucepan of water to the boil over high heat. Add ¼ teaspoon of the salt.

Add the mangetout to the boiling water and cook until bright green yet still crisp, about 1 minute. Remove the mangetout from the boiling water using a slotted spoon, transfer to a colander, and immediately rinse with cold water until cooled. Keep the water boiling.

Line a rimmed baking sheet with kitchen paper and spread the mangetout onto the baking sheet. Pat dry and set aside.

Set up an ice bath by placing about 1.5 liters ice and 500 ml of cold water in a large bowl.

Add the prawns to the boiling water. Cover the pan, turn off the heat, and let the prawns cook for 1 minute or until they are opaque and slightly pink.

Using a slotted spoon, transfer the prawns to the ice bath and let sit for 5 minutes to cool. Cut the prawns in half lengthwise.

Combine the lime zest, juice, oil, chilies, shallot, and remaining ¼ teaspoon salt in a large bowl and stir. Add the cooled prawns to the lime juice mixture, toss to combine, cover, and refrigerate for at least 30 minutes to marinate.

When ready to serve, add the mangetout, jicama, and coriander to the prawn mixture, and toss to combine. Divide among four serving plates and serve immediately.

Nutritional analysis per serving: *Calories: 330, Fat: 16 g, Saturated Fat: 2 g, Cholesterol: 215 mg, Fiber: 4 g, Protein: 27 g, Carbohydrates: 20 g, Sodium: 660 mg*

Niçoise Salad with Poached Salmon

There is nothing I enjoy more than sharing a meal with friends and family, especially on the weekend. Sunday brunch is a great time to connect with the people you love, and this salad is easy to make, satisfying, and delicious for those special moments.

Serves: 4
Prep Time: 25 minutes
Cook Time: 20 minutes

- 4 large omega-3 eggs
- 250 g frozen artichoke hearts, thawed
- 225 g French beans, trimmed
- 1 lemon, thinly sliced
- 3 to 4 parsley sprigs
- 4 (115- to 175-g) boneless, skin-on wild salmon fillets
- sea salt and freshly ground black pepper
- 5 oil-packed anchovy fillets
- 2 tablespoons anchovy oil or extra-virgin olive oil
- 1½ tablespoons cider vinegar
- 8 to 10 soft lettuce leaves
- 450 g cherry or baby plum tomatoes, halved
- 4 tablespoons Kalamata olives, pitted

Put the eggs in a large saucepan and add enough cold water to cover by 2.5 cm. Bring the water to the boil over medium heat, remove from the heat, and cover. Let stand for 12 minutes. Transfer the eggs to a bowl using a slotted spoon and cover with cold water. When the eggs have cooled, peel them and cut them into halves. Set aside.

Bring the water back to the boil over medium heat. Add the artichoke hearts and cook until tender, about 5 minutes. Using a slotted spoon, transfer the artichoke hearts to a small bowl. Add the French beans to the boiling water and cook until tender, 2 to 3 minutes. Prepare a water bath while the beans cook by filling a bowl with half ice cubes and half cold water. Drain the beans and add them to the water bath.

Pour 2.5 cm of water into a large frying pan, along with the lemon slices and parsley. Bring the water to the boil over high heat. Season the salmon fillets with a pinch of salt and gently add them, skin-side down, to the water. Cover, reduce the heat to medium, and cook to the desired doneness, about 8 minutes. Carefully remove the salmon from the water and set aside.

Finely dice one of the anchovies and place in a small bowl. Add the oil, vinegar, ¼ teaspoon salt, and ½ teaspoon black pepper and whisk to combine all of the ingredients.

Line a large platter with lettuce leaves and top with the artichoke hearts, French beans, eggs, tomatoes, olives, and the remaining 4 anchovy fillets. Pour the dressing over the vegetables on the platter. Place the poached salmon on top of the salad and serve.

Nutritional analysis per serving: Calories: 251, Fat: 17 g, Saturated Fat: 3 g, Cholesterol: 228 mg, Fiber: 7 g, Protein: 12 g, Carbohydrates: 16 g, Sodium: 564 mg

Salmon Salad Wraps

When you trade a less nutritious food for a higher-quality food without losing the personality of the dish, I call it a "swap." In this recipe, swap that blood-sugar-spiking flour tortilla for crisp lettuce to enjoy a low-glycemic meal that satisfies both your taste buds and your waistline.

Serves: 4
Prep Time: 20 minutes
Cook Time: 5 minutes

- 1 teaspoon sea salt
- juice of 1 lemon
- 2 (225-g) boneless, skinless wild salmon fillets
- 1 large yellow pepper, seeded and finely chopped
- ¼ small red onion, finely chopped
- 1 tablespoon finely chopped jalapeño chili
- 1 tablespoon rinsed capers, finely chopped
- 3 tablespoons fresh lime juice
- 1 tablespoon extra-virgin olive oil
- 2 tablespoons finely chopped fresh coriander
- 12 crisp lettuce leaves
- 2 avocados, stoned, peeled, and sliced

In a large frying pan, bring 1.5 liters of water and ½ teaspoon of the salt to the boil over high heat. Add the lemon juice. Gently slide the salmon fillets into the boiling water. Reduce to a low simmer and poach until the salmon is cooked through and opaque, about 5 minutes. Remove from the water and set aside to cool to room temperature, 5 to 10 minutes. When cooled, flake into small pieces.

Meanwhile, in a large bowl, combine the yellow pepper, onion, chili, capers, lime juice, oil, and remaining ½ teaspoon salt and mix well. Let the salad stand while the salmon cooks and cools. Then gently fold the salmon and coriander into the salad.

Divide the lettuce leaves among four serving plates. Then divide the salmon mixture into 12 portions and spoon a portion onto each leaf. Top the salmon mixture with the sliced avocado, fold the lettuce around the salmon and avocado to form a wrap, and then serve seam-side down.

Nutritional analysis per serving: *Calories: 370, Fat: 26 g, Saturated Fat: 4 g, Cholesterol: 60 mg, Fiber: 8 g, Protein: 25 g, Carbohydrates: 14 g, Sodium: 550 mg*

SEAWEED SALAD WITH POACHED PRAWNS

You can substitute 450 g of squid for the prawns. Buy it cleaned, then cut the bodies into 5-mm-thick rings and the tentacles in half lengthwise. Cook just until the tentacles curl and stiffen, about 30 seconds. Drain and immediately rinse under cold water until cool.

Serves: 4
Prep Time: 10 minutes
Cook Time: 3 minutes

- 225 g shredded dried wakame seaweed
- 225 g shredded dried kombu seaweed
- 450 g large raw prawns, peeled and deveined
- 3 tablespoons gluten-free, low-sodium tamari
- 2 tablespoons apple cider vinegar
- 1 tablespoon toasted sesame oil
- 1 teaspoon freshly grated horseradish
- 2 celery stalks, thinly sliced
- 1 spring onion, thinly sliced
- 1 tablespoon roasted sesame seeds
- 2 avocados, stoned, peeled, and sliced

Place the seaweeds in a large bowl and add enough cold water to cover by 7 cm. Let stand until just softened, about 10 minutes. Drain well.

Bring a medium saucepan of water to the boil over high heat. Add the prawns and cook until just opaque throughout, about 3 minutes. Drain and rinse under cold water until cool.

In a separate large bowl, combine the tamari, vinegar, sesame oil, and horseradish and mix well. Stir in the seaweed, celery, spring onion, and cooled prawns. Sprinkle with the sesame seeds.

Divide the salad among four plates, top with the sliced avocado, and serve.

Nutritional analysis per serving: *Calories: 320, Fat: 20 g, Saturated Fat: 3 g, Cholesterol: 145 mg, Fiber: 11 g, Protein: 20 g, Carbohydrates: 18 g, Sodium: 500 mg*

ALMOND CHICKEN SALAD

Radicchio, an Italian lettuce, adds beautiful color to this zesty salad.

Serves: 4
Prep Time: 20 minutes
Cook Time: 8 minutes

- 25 g flaked almonds
- 4 (115-g) thin-cut boneless, skinless chicken breasts
- 6 tablespoons extra-virgin olive oil
- ½ teaspoon sea salt
- grated zest and juice of 2 limes
- 2 small shallots, finely chopped
- 2 teaspoons chili powder
- 1 teaspoon paprika
- 1 head romaine lettuce, roughly torn
- 1 head radicchio, shredded
- ½ head Chinese leaves, shredded
- 2 carrots, peeled and shaved into strips

Preheat the oven to 230°C/Gas 8. Toast the almonds in a small frying pan over medium heat, stirring frequently, until golden brown.

Heat a well-seasoned griddle pan over high heat. Rub the chicken breasts with 2 tablespoons of the oil and season with ¼ teaspoon of the salt. Working in batches, place the chicken on the griddle pan and cook for 2 to 3 minutes per side. Transfer the chicken to a chopping board and let cool. Once cool, slice each chicken breast into strips.

In a small bowl, whisk together the remaining 4 tablespoons oil, lime zest and juice, shallots, chili powder, paprika, and remaining salt.

In a large bowl, combine the lettuce, radicchio, Chinese leaves, and carrots and toss with the vinaigrette to coat evenly. Arrange the warm chicken strips over the salad and garnish with toasted almonds. Serve.

Nutritional analysis per serving: *Calories: 435, Fat: 28 g, Saturated Fat: 4 g, Cholesterol: 109 mg, Fiber: 7 g, Protein: 38 g, Carbohydrates: 15 g, Sodium: 534 mg*

CAESAR SALAD WITH GRILLED CHICKEN

This version of Caesar salad uses a hard-boiled egg in the dressing instead of the classic raw egg yolk. The cooked egg whites, diced and added to the salad, add extra protein.

Serves: 4
Prep Time: 20 minutes
Cook Time: 15 minutes

- 4 (115- to 175-g) boneless, skinless chicken breasts or thighs
- 2 garlic cloves, 1 thinly sliced and 1 crushed
- 5 tablespoons extra-virgin olive oil
- ¼ teaspoon sea salt
- ¼ teaspoon freshly ground black pepper
- 1 large omega-3 egg
- 2 teaspoons Dijon mustard
- ½ teaspoon anchovy paste
- ¼ teaspoon Worcestershire sauce
- 2 tablespoons fresh lemon juice
- 1 head romaine lettuce, cut into 5-cm-wide strips

In a large bowl, combine the chicken, sliced garlic, 1 tablespoon of the olive oil, the salt, and the black pepper. Cover and marinate for at least 15 minutes in the refrigerator.

Put the egg in a small saucepan and add enough cold water to cover by 2.5 cm. Bring to the boil over medium heat, remove from the heat, and cover. Let stand for 10 minutes. Using a slotted spoon, transfer the egg to a bowl and cover with cold water. When cooled, peel the egg. Separate the yolk from the white. Dice the white and set aside.

In a small bowl, use a fork to mash the egg yolk with the crushed garlic, Dijon mustard, anchovy paste, and Worcestershire sauce until well combined. Whisk in the lemon juice. Drizzle in the remaining 4 tablespoons oil, whisking as you drizzle, until the dressing is fully combined.

Heat a well-seasoned griddle pan or grill to medium-high. Grill the chicken until it is firm to the touch and cooked through, about 6 minutes per side (the internal temperature should reach 75°C), turning once during cooking. Transfer the chicken to a chopping board and let rest for 5 minutes. Thinly slice the chicken across the grain.

Place the lettuce in a large bowl, add the dressing, and toss well to coat evenly. Top with the sliced chicken, garnish with the diced egg white, and serve.

Nutritional analysis per serving: Calories: 330, Fat: 22 g, Saturated Fat: 3 g, Cholesterol: 129 mg, Fiber: 3 g, Protein: 28 g, Carbohydrates: 7 g, Sodium: 428 mg

CHICKEN SALAD IN CHICORY CUPS

This is a great way to use up leftover cooked chicken. If you don't have any cooked chicken on hand, grill or poach 450 g of boneless, skinless chicken breasts, cool, then cut into bite-size pieces.

Serves: 4
Prep Time: 20 minutes

- 1 avocado, peeled and stoned
- 4 tablespoons fresh parsley leaves, plus extra for garnish
- 4 tablespoons fresh mint leaves, plus extra for garnish
- 4 tablespoons fresh lemon juice
- 1 teaspoon anchovy paste
- sea salt and freshly ground black pepper
- 450 g cooked boneless, skinless chicken breasts, cut into 1-cm cubes
- 4 celery stalks, finely diced
- 1 shallot, finely chopped
- 2 heads chicory, leaves separated

In a food processor or blender, puree the avocado, parsley, mint, lemon juice, 2 tablespoons of water, anchovy paste, ½ teaspoon salt, and ¼ teaspoon black pepper until smooth. Transfer to a large bowl.

Add the chicken, celery, shallot, a pinch of salt, and ¼ teaspoon black pepper. Fold until well mixed.

To serve, divide the chicken salad among the chicory leaves (approximately 10 per person) and garnish with additional parsley and mint.

Nutritional analysis per serving: *Calories: 260, Fat: 11 g, Saturated Fat: 1.5 g, Cholesterol: 65 mg, Fiber: 12 g, Protein: 25 g, Carbohydrates: 19 g, Sodium: 550 mg*

Pan-Roasted Chicken Thighs with Celery Salad and Mustard Vinaigrette

Prepare this hearty salad a few hours ahead of time and store it in the fridge.

Serves: 4
Prep Time: 20 minutes
Cook Time: 20 minutes

- 2 anchovy fillets, finely chopped
- 1½ tablespoons fresh lemon juice
- 1 teaspoon Dijon mustard
- 1½ teaspoons celery seeds
- 3 tablespoons extra-virgin olive oil
- 450 g celery hearts with leaves, thinly sliced
- 10 to 12 large radishes (about 200 g), sliced
- 3 spring onions, chopped
- 1 tablespoon coconut oil
- 450 g boneless, skinless chicken thighs
- ¼ teaspoon sea salt and ¼ teaspoon freshly ground black pepper

In a small bowl, combine the chopped anchovies, lemon juice, mustard, and 1 teaspoon of the celery seeds. Whisk in the olive oil to emulsify.

In a large bowl, combine the celery, radishes, and spring onions. Drizzle the dressing over the salad and toss.

In a large nonstick sauté pan, warm the coconut oil over medium-high heat until shimmering. Season the chicken thighs with the salt and black pepper. Add the chicken to the pan and sauté, turning occasionally, until fully cooked, 16 to 18 minutes, depending on thickness. Cut into one of the thickest chicken thighs to check for doneness; the internal temperature should be 75°C and the juices should run clear. Remove the chicken from the pan and sprinkle with the remaining ½ teaspoon celery seeds. To serve, divide the salad among four plates and top with a chicken thigh.

Nutritional analysis per serving: *Calories: 280, Fat: 19 g, Saturated Fat: 6 g, Cholesterol: 110 mg, Fiber: 3 g, Protein: 23 g, Carbohydrates: 6 g, Sodium: 400 mg*

WALDORF SALAD WITH SMOKED PAPRIKA

Most commercial mayonnaise on the market is laden with preservatives, additives, and even sweeteners that are not necessary and thus make mayo a junk food. Make your own mayo from organic omega-3 eggs (see page 299; it's easier than you think!) or try Vegenaise, an eggless "mayo" made from rapeseed oil.

Serves: 4
Prep Time: 30 minutes, plus chilling time
Cook Time: 10 minutes

- 1 teaspoon dried rosemary
- 1 teaspoon dried thyme
- ½ teaspoon sea salt
- ½ teaspoon freshly ground black pepper
- 450 g thin-cut boneless, skinless chicken breasts
- 2 large celery stalks with leaves, thinly sliced
- 2 spring onions, chopped
- 1 red pepper, seeded and chopped
- 75 g chopped walnuts
- 3 tablespoons Mayonnaise (page 299) or Vegenaise
- 1 tablespoon fresh lemon juice
- 1 teaspoon smoked paprika
- 150 g mixed salad leaves

Fill a frying pan with 5 cm of water. Add the rosemary, thyme, and ¼ teaspoon each of the salt and black pepper and bring to the boil over high heat. Add the chicken. Cover, reduce the heat to medium, and cook until done, about 10 minutes. Transfer the chicken breasts to a bowl and let them cool. Reserve 2 tablespoons of the cooking liquid.

Cut or shred the cooled chicken into small pieces. Add the celery, spring onions, red pepper, and walnuts to the chicken.

In a small bowl, whisk together the reserved poaching liquid, mayonnaise, lemon juice, paprika, and the remaining ¼ teaspoon each salt and black pepper. Add the dressing to the chicken mixture, stirring to combine. Cover and refrigerate for 2 to 3 hours to allow the flavors to mingle.

To serve, divide the salad leaves among four plates and top with the chicken salad.

Nutritional analysis per serving: *Calories: 320, Fat: 21 g, Saturated Fat: 2.5 g, Cholesterol: 75 mg, Fiber: 3 g, Protein: 28 g, Carbohydrates: 7 g, Sodium: 510 mg*

Tandoori Lettuce Cups with Cumin Sauce

This is a hearty meal packed with healing spices that cool inflammation throughout the body. Don't let the lettuce deceive you—you will be energized and satisfied for hours after enjoying this Indian dish.

Serves: 6
Prep Time: 25 minutes, plus marinating time
Cook Time: 20 minutes

- 2 tablespoons fresh lemon juice
- 4 spring onions, thinly sliced
- 3 tablespoons chopped fresh root ginger
- 1 tablespoon paprika
- 2½ teaspoons ground cumin
- ½ teaspoon sea salt
- ¼ teaspoon cayenne pepper
- 900 g boneless, skinless chicken thighs, cut into 4-cm pieces
- 2 to 3 tablespoons extra-virgin olive oil
- 1 red pepper, seeded and cut into 1-cm-thick strips
- 1 yellow pepper, seeded and cut into 1-cm-thick strips
- 1 small red onion, halved and thinly sliced
- 120 ml Mayonnaise (page 299) or Vegenaise
- grated zest and juice of 1 lime
- 1 small head round lettuce, leaves separated
- coriander sprigs, for garnish

In a large bowl, combine the lemon juice, spring onions, ginger, paprika, 2 teaspoons of the cumin, ¼ teaspoon of the salt, and the cayenne and mix well. Add the chicken and toss to coat. Cover and marinate for at least 20 minutes and up to 2½ hours in the refrigerator.

Heat a well-seasoned griddle pan over medium–high heat. Brush with 1 tablespoon of the oil. Remove the chicken from the marinade and grill the chicken, turning occasionally, until no longer pink in the center, 8 to

10 minutes. Work in batches if necessary, adding more oil to the pan if needed. Transfer the cooked chicken to a plate.

Meanwhile, preheat the grill. On a large rimmed baking sheet, toss the peppers and onion with the remaining 1 tablespoon oil. Grill until fork-tender, 12 to 15 minutes, tossing once to ensure even cooking.

In a small bowl, whisk together the mayonnaise, lime zest and juice, remaining ½ teaspoon cumin, and remaining ¼ teaspoon salt.

To serve, have guests wrap chicken and vegetables in lettuce leaves and top with cumin sauce and coriander sprigs.

Nutritional analysis per serving: *Calories: 400, Fat: 28 g, Saturated Fat: 4.5 g, Cholesterol: 150 mg, Fiber: 1 g, Protein: 30 g, Carbohydrates: 5 g, Sodium: 430 mg*

Chicken Satay with Cucumber Salad

Sesame-Coconut Curry Sauce is the perfect accompaniment for these Thai-inspired chicken skewers, and the cucumber salad provides a cool, crisp crunch. You will need eight wooden or bamboo skewers for this recipe; soak them in warm water for at least 15 minutes before cooking so that they don't burn.

Serves: 4
Prep Time: 25 minutes
Cook Time: 15 minutes

- 1 tablespoon Thai fish sauce or gluten-free, low-sodium tamari
- 1 tablespoon plus 2 teaspoons fresh lime juice
- 1 large shallot, finely chopped
- 2 garlic cloves, crushed
- 1 teaspoon finely chopped fresh root ginger
- ¼ teaspoon ground turmeric
- 675 g boneless, skinless chicken thighs, cut into 2.5-cm-thick strips
- 225 g green beans, trimmed and halved
- 1 small cucumber, peeled, halved lengthwise, and thinly sliced
- ½ small red onion, thinly sliced
- 2 teaspoons extra-virgin olive oil, plus extra if needed for baking sheet
- ¼ teaspoon toasted sesame oil
- ¼ teaspoon sea salt
- Sesame-Coconut Curry Sauce (page 291)

Preheat the oven to 230°C/Gas 8, or heat a grill or well-seasoned griddle pan over medium-high heat.

In a large bowl, whisk together the Thai fish sauce, 1 tablespoon of the lime juice, the shallot, garlic, ginger, and turmeric. Add the chicken and toss to coat. Place the chicken in the refrigerator to marinate for 10 minutes.

Meanwhile, pour 250 ml of water into the bottom of a medium saucepan and bring it to the boil over high heat. Place a steaming rack or basket over the boiling water. Add the green beans, cover, and steam until bright green and crisp-tender, 4 to 5 minutes.

Transfer the green beans to a medium bowl. Add the cucumber, onion, remaining 2 teaspoons lime juice, olive oil, sesame oil, and salt and toss well to combine.

Thread the chicken strips onto the skewers, allowing them to bunch up slightly and covering as much skewer as possible. Leave just the tip and end of the skewers exposed.

If using the oven, lay the skewers on a lightly oiled baking sheet and roast, turning once, until cooked through, 10 to 15 minutes, or grill for 2 to 3 minutes on each side.

Serve the satay with the cucumber salad. Offer the curry sauce alongside for dipping.

Nutritional analysis per serving: *Calories: 260, Fat: 10 g, Saturated Fat: 2 g, Cholesterol: 160 mg, Fiber: 2 g, Protein: 35 g, Carbohydrates: 8 g, Sodium: 575 mg*

THAI CHICKEN SALAD

If you're in a hurry, leftover cooked chicken works great in this salad; just skip the poaching step. The poaching liquid makes a delicious soup base, though. Let it cool and store it in the refrigerator for up to 3 days or in the freezer for up to 6 months.

Serves: 4
Prep Time: 15 minutes
Cook Time: 10 minutes

- 1 liter low-sodium chicken stock
- 8 thin slices peeled fresh root ginger
- 3 garlic cloves, halved
- 1 large spring onion, cut into 5-cm pieces
- ½ teaspoon sea salt
- 2 boneless, skinless chicken breasts, cut into 2.5-cm pieces
- 2 tablespoons extra-virgin olive oil
- 1 tablespoon fresh lime juice
- 1 tablespoon Thai fish sauce
- pinch of crushed chili flakes
- 1 medium head Chinese leaves or green cabbage, shredded
- ¼ red onion or 1 large shallot, thinly sliced
- ½ large cucumber, thinly sliced
- 4 plum tomatoes, cut into 8 wedges
- 25 g roughly chopped mixed fresh herbs, such as coriander, mint, and/or basil
- 2 tablespoons flaked or sliced almonds

In a medium saucepan, combine the chicken stock, ginger, garlic, spring onion, and salt. Bring to a gentle simmer over medium heat, then add the chicken. Cover the pan, turn the heat to the lowest setting, and simmer for 8 minutes. Turn off the heat and let the chicken sit in the liquid for 2 more minutes, then transfer the chicken to a plate to cool. (Save the poaching liquid for another use, if desired.)

While the chicken poaches and cools, whisk together the olive oil, lime juice, fish sauce, and chili flakes in a large bowl. When the chicken is cool, gently pull it apart into large shreds, add it to the dressing, and toss.

Add the Chinese leaves, onion, cucumber, and tomatoes to the bowl. Toss to combine well. Top with the herbs and almonds and serve.

Nutritional analysis per serving: Calories: 220, Fat: 12 g, Saturated Fat: 2 g, Cholesterol: 65 mg, Fiber: 2 g, Protein: 21 g, Carbohydrates: 6 g, Sodium: 564 mg

CHINESE CHICKEN SALAD

This lemon-scented salad brightens the palate and awakens your senses. Choose a lemon with a thin skin, bright yellow color, and a slightly tender touch.

Serves: 4
Prep Time: 20 minutes
Cook Time: 20 minutes

- 1 large head Chinese leaves, shredded
- 1 large daikon radish (mooli), peeled and grated
- 1 large carrot, peeled and grated
- 50 g sugar snap peas, sliced
- 2 spring onions, finely chopped
- 1½ tablespoons extra-virgin olive oil
- 1 tablespoon fresh lemon juice
- 2 teaspoons gluten-free, low-sodium tamari
- ½ teaspoon grated fresh lemon zest
- 4 (115-g) boneless, skinless chicken thighs
- ¼ teaspoon sea salt
- ¼ teaspoon freshly ground black pepper
- 1 tablespoon coconut oil
- 1 to 2 teaspoons sesame seeds

In a large bowl, combine the Chinese leaves, daikon radish, carrot, sugar snap peas, and spring onions. Add the olive oil, lemon juice, tamari, and lemon zest and toss to combine.

Season the chicken with the salt and black pepper. In a large nonstick pan, warm the coconut oil over medium-high heat. Sauté the chicken until golden brown and cooked through (the internal temperature should reach 75°C), 8 to 10 minutes per side.

Divide the salad between four plates and top with the chicken. Garnish with sesame seeds and serve.

Nutritional analysis per serving: *Calories: 243, Fat: 14 g, Saturated Fat: 5 g, Cholesterol: 108 mg, Fiber: 2 g, Protein: 24 g, Carbohydrates: 5 g, Sodium: 387 mg*

Chicken Yakitori with Chinese Cabbage Slaw

Yakitori is simply Japanese for small, bite-size pieces of chicken (or other meat) that have been skewered, marinated, and grilled. Once you try this dish and experience firsthand how simple and tasty this style of cooking can be, you will return to this recipe time and time again. You will need eight wooden or bamboo skewers for this recipe; soak them in warm water for at least 15 minutes before cooking so that they don't burn.

Serves: 4
Prep Time: 20 minutes
Cook Time: 10 minutes

- 1 tablespoon gluten-free, low-sodium tamari
- 2 teaspoons toasted sesame oil
- 2 teaspoons fresh lemon or lime juice
- 1 teaspoon grated fresh root ginger
- 675 g boneless, skinless chicken thighs, cut into 2.5-cm-thick pieces
- 225 g green beans, trimmed and halved
- 1 large head Chinese leaves, finely shredded
- 4 large radishes, halved and thinly sliced
- 1½ tablespoons extra-virgin olive oil, plus more if needed for baking sheet
- ¼ teaspoon sea salt
- 8 large chestnut or button mushrooms, trimmed and quartered
- 1 small courgette, halved lengthwise and cut crosswise into 5-mm-thick slices

Preheat the oven to 230°C/Gas 8, or heat a grill or well-seasoned griddle pan over medium-high heat.

In a large bowl, combine the tamari, 1 teaspoon of the sesame oil, 1 teaspoon of the citrus juice, and the ginger and mix well. Add the chicken and place in the refrigerator to marinate for 10 minutes.

Meanwhile, pour 250 ml of water into the bottom of a medium saucepan and bring it to the boil over high heat. Place a steaming rack or basket over the boiling water. Add the green beans, cover, and steam until bright green and crisp-tender, 4 to 5 minutes. Transfer the beans to a large bowl.

Add the Chinese leaves and radishes to the beans, then add 1 table-spoon of the olive oil, the salt, the remaining 1 teaspoon sesame oil, and the remaining 1 teaspoon citrus juice. Toss the slaw well and set aside.

Thread the chicken, mushrooms, and courgette slices onto the skewers, bunching up the chicken slightly to keep it compact. Try to fill up most of each skewer, leaving only a little wood exposed at each end.

If using the oven, lay the skewers on a lightly oiled baking sheet and brush the mushrooms and courgettes with the remaining ½ tablespoon olive oil. Roast, turning once, until cooked through, about 8 minutes, or grill for 2 to 3 minutes on each side.

Divide the slaw among four plates and serve with two skewers on each.

Nutritional analysis per serving: *Calories: 300, Fat: 13 g, Saturated Fat: 2.5 g, Cholesterol: 160 mg, Fiber: 3 g, Protein: 36 g, Carbohydrates: 9 g, Sodium: 490 mg*

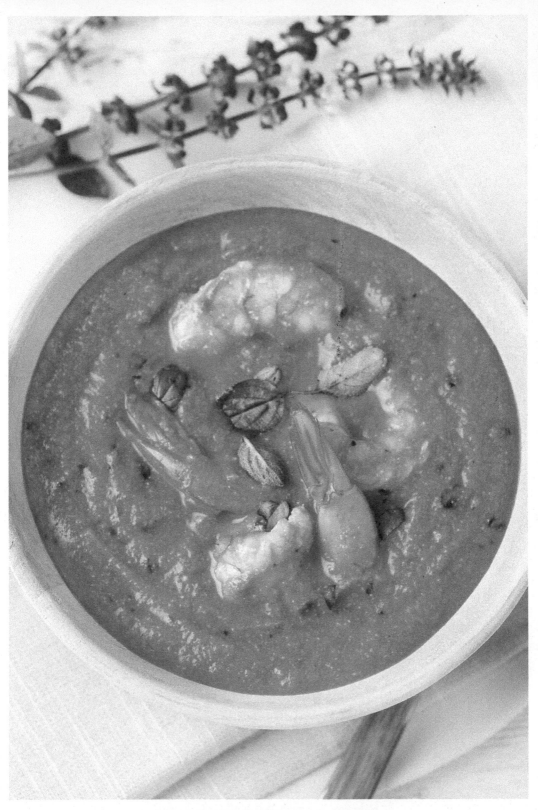

Tomato–Basil Soup with Shrimp (page 128)

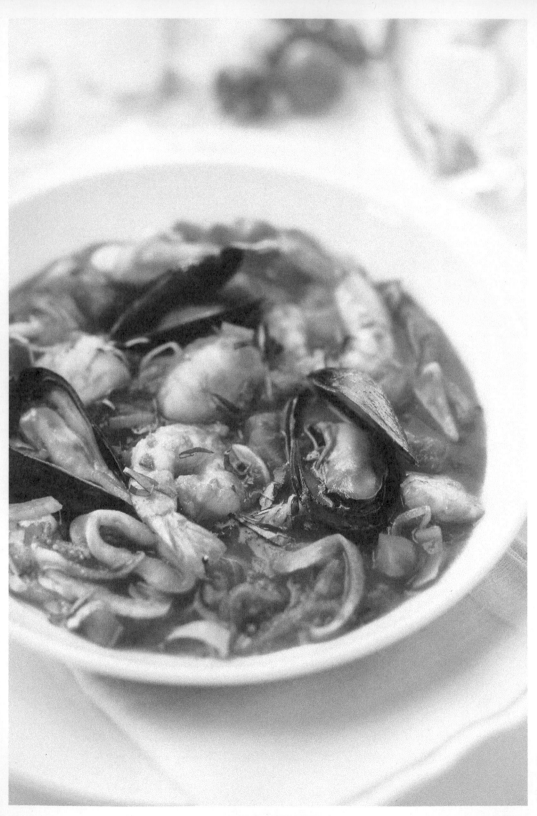

Cioppino (page 139)

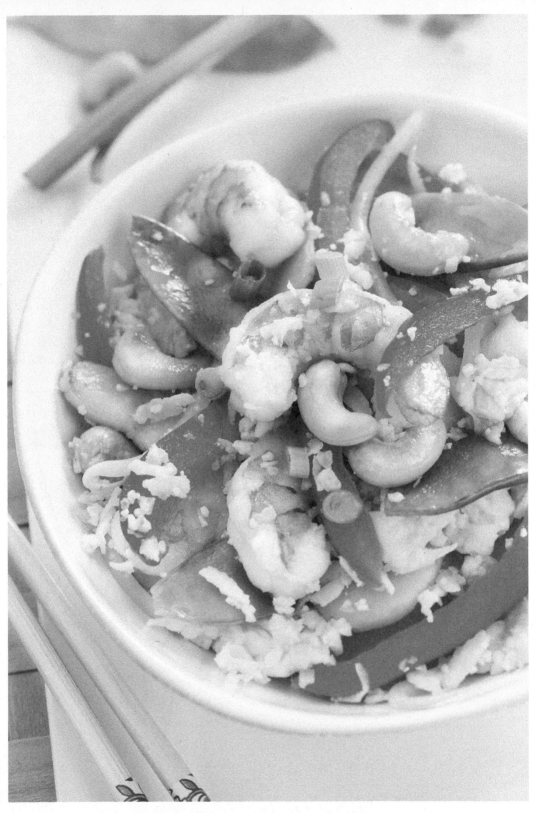

Fried "Rice" with Prawns (page 148)

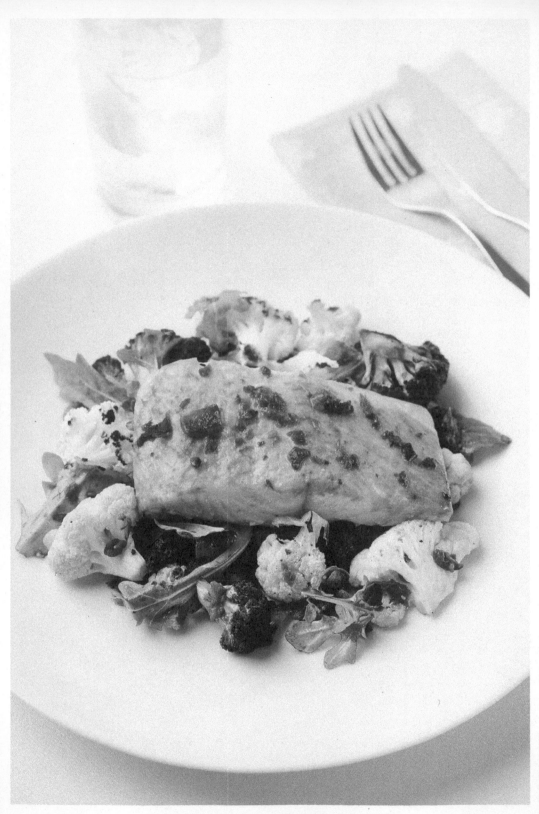

Chipotle Salmon with Rocket Salad (page 160)

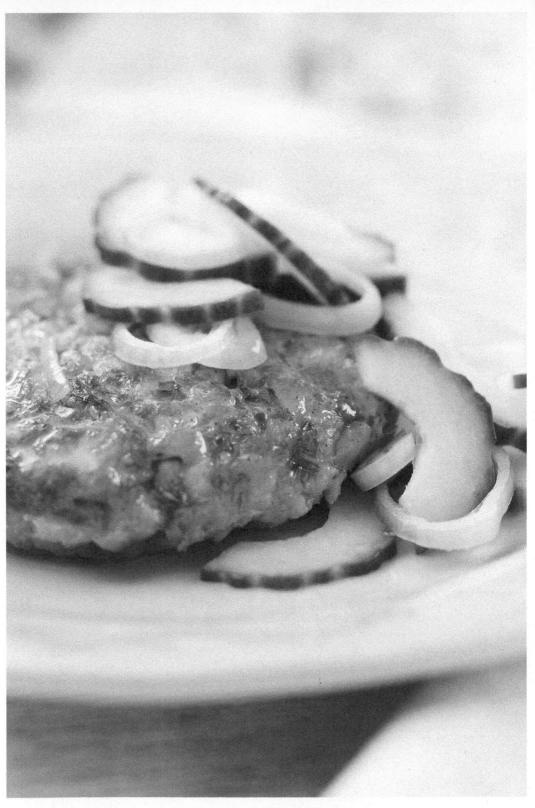

Asian-Spiced Salmon Cakes (page 163)

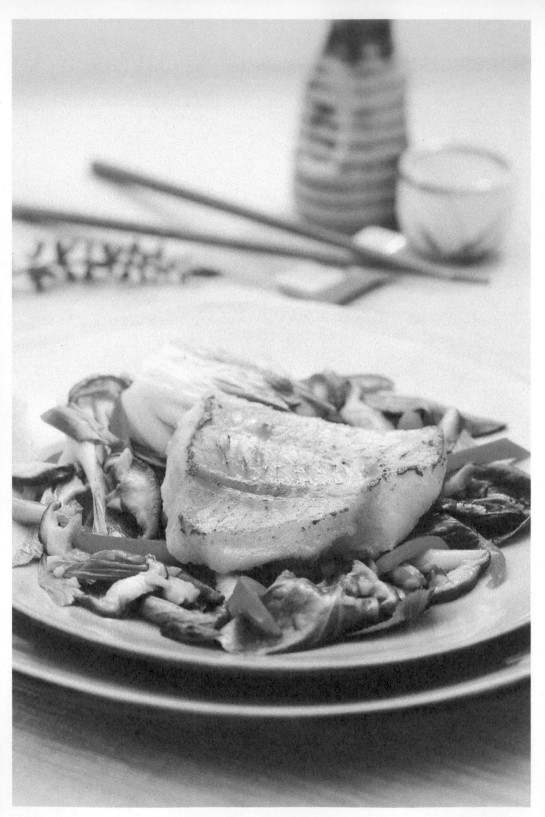

Pak Choi Stir-Fry with Black Cod (page 168)

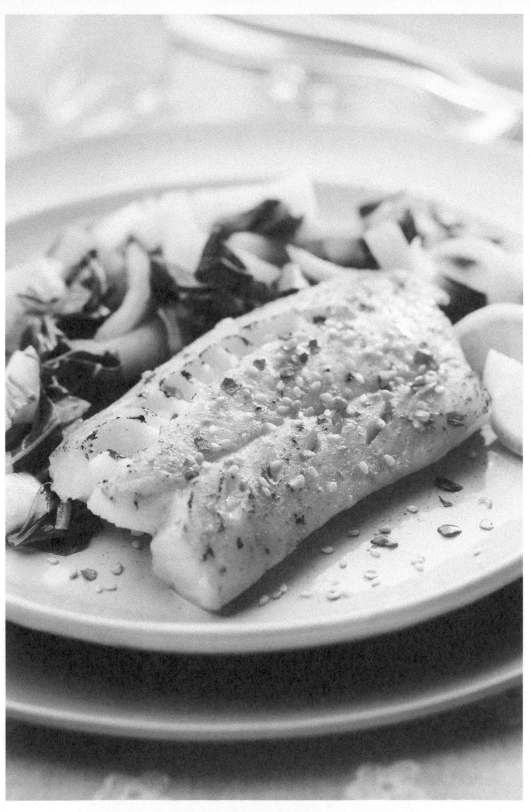

Miso-Marinated Cod with Fresh Basil and Pak Choi (page 170)

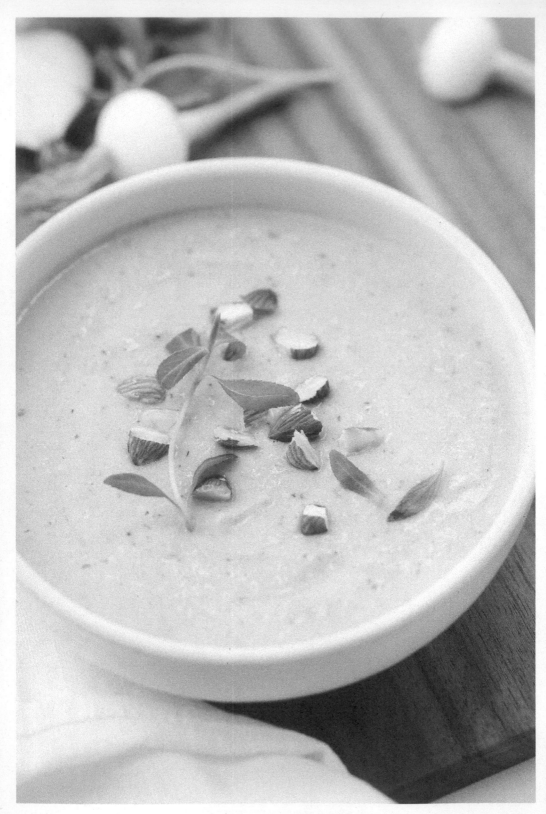

Onion-Leek Soup (page 126)

CHICKEN SPRING ROLLS WITH ALMOND SAUCE

This recipe introduces kelp noodles as an alternative to grain-based pasta. Kelp noodles are made from sea vegetables and are very low in carbohydrates. They can be found in the Asian section of some supermarkets. If you can't find them, feel free to use shirataki noodles, which are made from water and glucomannan fiber from the konjac root (you can typically find these in the refrigerated section where other vegetarian foods, such as tofu, tempeh, hummus, and miso, are kept).

Serves: 4
Prep Time: 15 minutes
Cook Time: 5 minutes

- 1½ teaspoons coconut oil
- 450 g chicken strips
- ¼ teaspoon sea salt
- ¼ teaspoon freshly ground black pepper
- 115 g almond butter
- 1 large spring onion, roughly chopped
- 1½ teaspoons coconut aminos
- ¼ teaspoon ground ginger
- 350 g kelp noodles or shirataki noodles, chopped
- 16 fresh mint leaves
- 16 soft lettuce leaves
- ¼ small red onion, thinly sliced
- ½ medium daikon radish (mooli), peeled and thinly sliced
- 1 medium red pepper, seeded and thinly sliced
- 75 g sliced hearts of palm, drained if canned

In a large nonstick sauté pan, warm the coconut oil over medium–high heat. Season the chicken with the salt and black pepper and add to the pan. Cook until the chicken is cooked through, about 2 minutes per side.

In a food processor, combine the almond butter, spring onion, coconut aminos, and ginger. Process, adding 4 to 5 tablespoons of hot water through the feed tube until the sauce reaches the desired consistency.

Place the noodles in a colander and rinse well. In a small bowl, mix the noodles with about half of the almond sauce, reserving the remaining sauce.

To make the spring rolls, place a mint leaf at the bottom of each lettuce leaf. Add a small amount of noodles, chicken, onion, daikon, red pepper, and hearts of palm. Top with a tablespoon of almond sauce. Repeat to make the remaining rolls. Serve.

Nutritional analysis per serving: Calories: 410, Fat: 23 g, Saturated Fat: 4.5 g, Cholesterol: 75 mg, Fiber: 6 g, Protein: 33 g, Carbohydrates: 20 g, Sodium: 480 mg

FENNEL AND CHERRY TOMATO SALAD WITH PORK FILLET

Choose pasture-raised, grass-fed pork from a local supplier, when possible, to avoid antibiotics typically used for animals raised in confinement.

Serves: 4
Prep Time: 20 minutes
Cook Time: 6 minutes

- 2 medium fennel bulbs, quartered and thinly sliced, plus 2 tablespoons chopped fennel fronds
- 900 g cherry tomatoes, halved
- 120 g jicama or daikon radish (mooli), finely sliced
- 1 large spring onion, finely chopped
- 1 teaspoon fennel seeds
- 2½ tablespoons extra-virgin olive oil
- 1 tablespoon fresh lemon juice
- sea salt and freshly ground black pepper
- ½ teaspoon dried rosemary
- 1 (450-g) pork fillet, cut into bite-size pieces

In a large bowl, combine the fennel slices and fronds, tomatoes, jicama, spring onion, fennel seeds, 2 tablespoons of the olive oil, the lemon juice, ¼ teaspoon salt, and a pinch of black pepper. Stir to combine.

Meanwhile, in a spice grinder, pulse the rosemary, ¼ teaspoon salt, and a pinch of black pepper. Firmly rub the pork fillet pieces with the rosemary seasoning.

Warm the remaining ½ tablespoon olive oil in a large nonstick pan over medium–high heat. Add the pork and sauté, stirring occasionally, until the pork is cooked through, 5 to 6 minutes.

Transfer the pork to the salad. Stir to combine and serve.

Nutritional analysis per serving: *Calories: 280, Fat: 15 g, Saturated Fat: 3 g, Cholesterol: 60 mg, Fiber: 7 g, Protein: 22 g, Carbohydrates: 18 g, Sodium: 420 mg*

Taco Salad with Skirt Steak

The ground coriander and cayenne make this dish pop. Coriander is a slightly sweet spice and the cayenne has a nice amount of heat—both complement the citrus in this steak salad and make you feel as though you are at a Mexican fiesta.

Serves: 4
Prep Time: 20 minutes
Cook Time: 15 minutes

- 1 bunch coriander, including stems
- 1 spring onion, thinly sliced
- 4 tablespoons extra-virgin olive oil
- 2 tablespoons Mayonnaise (page 299) or Vegenaise
- 2 teaspoons distilled vinegar
- grated zest and juice of ½ lime
- sea salt and freshly ground black pepper
- 1 (450-g) grass-fed skirt steak
- 1 teaspoon ground coriander
- ½ teaspoon cayenne pepper
- 2 large romaine lettuce hearts, halved lengthwise and thinly sliced
- 450 g cherry or baby plum tomatoes, halved
- 4 medium peppers (any color), seeded and thinly sliced into rings
- 1 avocado, stoned, peeled, and thinly sliced
- 2 tablespoons toasted pumpkin seeds
- lime wedges, for serving

In a blender, combine the coriander, 1 teaspoon of the sliced spring onion, the olive oil, mayonnaise, vinegar, lime zest and juice, 2 tablespoons of water, ½ teaspoon salt, and a pinch of black pepper. Puree until very smooth, 1 to 2 minutes, and set aside.

Heat a well-seasoned griddle pan over medium-high heat. Season the steak with ¼ teaspoon salt and ½ teaspoon black pepper. When the pan is very hot, cook the steak until charred, turning once, 12 to 15 minutes for medium-rare (about 55°C). Transfer the steak to a chopping board and immediately sprinkle both sides with the coriander and cayenne. Let stand for 10 minutes, then cut into bite-size pieces.

In a large bowl, toss the romaine with one-third of the dressing and divide among four plates. Arrange the tomatoes, peppers, avocado, and steak on top and drizzle with the remaining dressing. Sprinkle the pmpkin seeds and remaining sliced spring onion on top. Serve with lime wedges on the side.

Nutritional analysis per serving: *Calories: 468, Fat: 32 g, Saturated Fat: 6 g, Cholesterol: 72 mg, Fiber: 8 g, Protein: 30 g, Carbohydrates: 18 g, Sodium: 526 mg*

Onion-Leek Soup

If you can't find chervil, you can substitute 75 g chopped fresh parsley plus 40 g chopped fresh tarragon. To make this a vegetarian soup, simply replace the chicken stock with vegetable stock (such as the Vegetable-Herb Stock on page 304).

Serves: 4
Prep Time: 15 minutes
Cook Time: 20 minutes

- 2 tablespoons extra-virgin olive oil, plus more for serving
- 3 leeks, white parts only, halved lengthwise and thinly sliced crosswise
- 1 medium onion, quartered and very thinly sliced
- ¾ teaspoon sea salt
- ½ teaspoon freshly ground black pepper
- 1 liter low-sodium chicken stock
- 400 g non-GMO silken tofu, drained and quartered
- 115 g chopped fresh chervil, plus more for garnish
- 2 tablespoons chopped toasted almonds

Heat the oil in a large saucepan over medium heat. Add the leeks and onion and season with ½ teaspoon salt and ¼ teaspoon black pepper. Stir well and cover. Cook, stirring occasionally, until translucent, about 5 minutes.

Add the stock to the saucepan. Bring to the boil, then reduce the heat to low, and simmer, uncovered, until the leeks are very soft, about 10 minutes. Add the tofu and return to the boil. Turn off the heat and carefully transfer the soup to a blender (see Note). Add the chervil and the remaining ¼ teaspoon each salt and black pepper and blend until very smooth, 2 to 3 minutes. (Alternatively, you can use a stick blender to puree the soup right in the pan.)

Ladle the soup into four serving bowls and top each serving with chervil and almonds.

Note: Always be very careful when pureeing hot liquids in a blender. The heat from the liquid can cause the pressure in the blender to build up under the lid, and when the blender is turned on, the top can blow off and your hot soup will fly everywhere. Keep the lid vented by removing the small window insert from the middle of the blender lid; hold a towel over the open window to prevent splattering. Always start on the lowest speed possible.

Nutritional analysis per serving: Calories: 290, Fat: 13 g, Saturated Fat: 2 g, Cholesterol: 25 mg, Fiber: 5 g, Protein: 14 g, Carbohydrates: 31 g, Sodium: 600 mg

Tomato-Basil Soup with Prawns

One of my favorite culinary tricks for making creamy, comforting soups without dairy is substituting cashews for double cream or butter in recipes. Cashews are mild in flavor and lend a creaminess that you can't get from other nuts. They also happen to be quite hypoallergenic, which is helpful for those with tree nut allergies.

Serves: 4
Prep Time: 10 minutes
Cook Time: 30 minutes

- 140 g raw cashews
- 2 tablespoons extra-virgin olive oil
- 1 onion, diced
- 4 garlic cloves, sliced
- 1 celery stalk, diced
- 1 bay leaf
- 1 tablespoon tomato puree
- 850 ml passata
- 350 ml low-sodium chicken stock
- 4 tablespoons unsweetened almond milk
- ½ teaspoon sea salt
- 4 tablespoons fresh basil leaves, plus extra chopped basil for garnish
- 20 large cooked, peeled prawns
- freshly ground black pepper

Place the cashews in a small, heatproof bowl and cover with 500 ml of boiling water. Cover the bowl and allow the cashews to sit for 15 minutes, then drain and reserve the nuts.

While the cashews are soaking, heat the olive oil in a medium saucepan over medium heat. Add the onion, garlic, celery, and bay leaf to the pan and cook, stirring occasionally, until the vegetables are soft and beginning to brown, about 10 minutes.

Stir in the tomato puree and cook for 2 more minutes. Add the passata, chicken stock, almond milk, cashews, and salt. Bring to a simmer, then reduce the heat to medium-low and cook for 15 minutes.

Remove the bay leaf and transfer the hot soup to a blender, and very carefully puree the soup starting on low speed, making sure to vent the lid (see Note). Once the soup is pureed, add the basil and give it a quick final spin in the blender.

Divide the prawns among four soup bowls and ladle the soup into each bowl. Sprinkle a pinch of black pepper over each bowl of soup, garnish with chopped basil, and serve.

Note: Always be very careful when pureeing hot liquids in a blender. The heat from the liquid can cause the pressure in the blender to build up under the lid, and when the blender is turned on, the top can blow off and your hot soup will fly everywhere. Keep the lid vented by removing the small window insert from the middle of the blender lid; hold a towel over the open window to prevent splattering. Always start on the lowest speed possible.

Nutritional analysis per serving: *Calories: 360, Fat: 21 g, Saturated Fat: 3.5 g, Cholesterol: 55 mg, Fiber: 6 g, Protein: 16 g, Carbohydrates: 32 g, Sodium: 490 mg*

THAI CHICKEN NOODLE SOUP

Kelp noodles are simple to prepare and low-glycemic. Their neutral flavor makes them an easy, versatile addition to soups such as this one. For a more substantial meal, pair this with Rocket and Fennel Salad (see page 252).

Serves: 4
Prep Time: 15 minutes
Cook Time: 20 minutes

- 1 liter low-sodium chicken stock
- 1 (400-ml) can full-fat unsweetened coconut milk
- 1 onion, quartered and thinly sliced
- 2 lemongrass stalks, cut into 10-cm lengths and smashed
- 1 long red chili (such as Anaheim), seeded and thinly sliced
- 450 g boneless, skinless chicken breasts, cut into strips
- 100 g sugar snap peas, halved
- 450 g kelp noodles, rinsed and drained
- 75 g bean sprouts
- ½ teaspoon sea salt
- ½ bunch coriander, including stems, chopped
- lime wedges, for serving

Combine the chicken stock, coconut milk, and 350 ml of water in a large saucepan. Add the onion, lemongrass, and chili and bring to the boil over medium-high heat. Reduce the heat to low and simmer until the onion is translucent, about 10 minutes.

Add the chicken and sugar snap peas and poach until the chicken is just cooked through, about 5 minutes. Discard the lemongrass. Add the kelp noodles and bean sprouts and cook until the noodles are just soft, about 2 minutes. Stir in the salt.

Divide the soup among four serving bowls and top with the coriander. Serve with the lime wedges.

Nutritional analysis per serving: Calories: 440, Fat: 25 g, Saturated Fat: 19 g, Cholesterol: 100 mg, Fiber: 4 g, Protein: 35 g, Carbohydrates: 21 g, Sodium: 490 mg

DINNER

Vegetarian and Vegan

BROCCOLI TOFU

It seems wherever I go, people ask me whether broccoli is good for thyroid health. When you cook broccoli just enough, you remove the goitrogenic compounds called thiocyanates. While thiocyanates are important for disease prevention and overall health, there is no research showing that they interfere with thyroid health. This recipe is one of my favorite ways to show people how to prepare broccoli for nutritional health as well as flavor and enjoyment.

Serves: 6
Prep Time: 20 minutes, plus draining time
Cook Time: 15 minutes

- 800 g non-GMO extra-firm tofu
- 1 teaspoon sea salt
- 675 g broccoli, stems peeled and cut into 5-mm-thick rounds, florets separated into bite-size pieces
- 4 tablespoons extra-virgin olive oil
- 4 tablespoons gluten-free, low-sodium tamari
- ¼ teaspoon crushed chili flakes
- 4 garlic cloves, thinly sliced
- 1 (225-g) can sliced water chestnuts, drained
- 75 g roasted cashews, coarsely chopped

Drain the tofu by placing the two blocks of tofu side by side on a rimmed baking sheet lined with several layers of kitchen paper. Top with additional kitchen paper and another baking sheet, and set something heavy, such as some canned goods, on the top baking sheet to help press out the liquid. Allow the tofu to drain for at least 30 minutes, changing the paper at least once. Cut the tofu into 2.5-cm cubes and set aside. Discard the wet kitchen paper from the baking sheet and apply new dry ones; set aside.

Bring a 5-liter saucepan of water to the boil over high heat. Add ½ teaspoon of the salt. Cook the broccoli stems and florets until bright green, 1 to 2 minutes. Drain the broccoli in a colander and rinse with cold water, tossing until cool. Dry thoroughly and set aside.

In a large nonstick frying pan, heat 2 tablespoons of the oil over medium-high heat until shimmering. Add the tofu and cook until golden brown, 2 to 3 minutes on each side. Once the tofu is browned, transfer it to the lined baking sheet. Reserve the oil in the pan.

In a small bowl whisk together the tamari, 4 tablespoons of water, the chili flakes, and the remaining ½ teaspoon salt and set aside.

Add the remaining 2 tablespoons oil to the pan and heat over high heat until shimmering. Add the broccoli, garlic, and water chestnuts and cook for 5 to 7 minutes, tossing often to avoid burning the garlic. Whisk the tamari sauce again and add it to the pan, along with the tofu, and toss to coat as the sauce thickens, about 1 minute more. Serve, topped with cashews.

Nutritional analysis per serving: Calories: 330, Fat: 22 g, Saturated Fat: 3.5 g, Cholesterol: 0 mg, Fiber: 6 g, Protein: 20 g, Carbohydrates: 16 g, Sodium: 432 mg

ROASTED VEGETABLE LASAGNE WITH CASHEW "RICOTTA"

Who says you can't enjoy comfort food while nourishing your body? Prepare this dish when you want to share a hearty, delicious meal the entire family will love. From my experience, it is best to double the recipe, making two lasagnes and freezing one for later, because this will quickly become a family favorite!

Serves: 6
Prep Time: 30 minutes
Cook Time: 55 minutes

- 1 small aubergine, very thinly sliced lengthwise
- 1 green courgette, very thinly sliced lengthwise
- 1 yellow courgette, very thinly sliced lengthwise
- 1 pepper (any color), seeded and cut into large squares
- 4 tablespoons extra-virgin olive oil
- 1 teaspoon sea salt
- 500 ml Cashew "Ricotta Cheese" (page 295)
- 1 large omega-3 egg, beaten
- ½ teaspoon dried oregano
- pinch of freshly ground black pepper
- 1 (425-g) can chopped tomatoes

Preheat the oven to 200°C/Gas 6.

In a large bowl, combine the aubergine, courgettes, and pepper with the oil and salt and toss well. Spread the vegetables in a single layer on two baking sheets and roast until they start to brown and caramelize around the edges, 20 to 25 minutes, rotating the sheets halfway through the cooking time.

Remove the baking sheets from the oven and set them aside to cool. Lower the oven temperature to 180°C/Gas 4.

While the vegetables are cooling, whisk together the cashew "cheese," egg, oregano, and black pepper in a medium bowl. Spread one-quarter of the mixture in the bottom of a 23-cm square glass baking dish, then spoon about a quarter of the chopped tomatoes on top. Cover the tomatoes with a layer of one of the types of vegetables. Continue to layer the remaining "cheese," tomatoes, and vegetables until everything is used up, finishing with tomatoes.

Bake the lasagne for 30 minutes. Allow it to cool for 5 minutes before serving.

Nutritional analysis per serving: Calories: 440, Fat: 34 g, Saturated Fat: 6 g, Cholesterol: 40 mg, Fiber: 6 g, Protein: 12 g, Carbohydrates: 28 g, Sodium: 512 mg

COCONUT CURRY WITH TOFU

The jalapeños make this curry nice and spicy. For a milder version, use only 2 jalapeños, and remove the seeds.

Serves: 4
Prep Time: 20 minutes
Cook Time: 30 minutes

- 1 small bunch coriander
- grated zest of 1 lime
- 3 jalapeño chilies, seeded if desired
- 2 garlic cloves, halved
- 2.5-cm piece fresh root ginger, peeled and roughly chopped
- 1 teaspoon ground coriander
- 1 teaspoon sea salt
- ½ teaspoon freshly ground black pepper
- ½ teaspoon ground cumin
- 1 (400-ml) can full-fat unsweetened coconut milk, chilled in the refrigerator overnight or for 12 hours
- 400 g non-GMO firm tofu, drained and cut into 1-cm cubes
- ½ small head cabbage, cut into 2.5-cm pieces
- 1 large head broccoli, florets cut into 2.5-cm pieces
- 1 large cauliflower, cored, florets cut into 2.5-cm pieces
- lime wedges, for serving

Trim the coriander leaves from the stems and reserve the leaves for garnish. Put the stems in a food processor and add the lime zest, jalapeños, garlic, ginger, ground coriander, ½ teaspoon of the salt, the black pepper, and the cumin. Pulse, scraping the sides of the bowl occasionally, until a smooth green curry paste forms.

Spoon 3 tablespoons of thick cream from the top of the can of coconut milk into a large saucepan. Cook over medium heat, stirring, until the oil separates and sizzles, about 1 minute. Add the green curry paste and cook, stirring, until thickened and nearly dry, about 2 minutes. Add the remaining coconut milk and 250 ml water. Bring to the boil. Add the tofu and return to the boil, then reduce the heat to low and simmer for about 20 minutes.

Meanwhile, bring a large saucepan of water to the boil. Add ¼ teaspoon of the salt to the water. Add the cabbage and cook until the thick white parts are just tender, about 3 minutes. Transfer the cabbage to the curry with a slotted spoon. Add the broccoli and cauliflower to the boiling water. Cook until crisp-tender, about 4 minutes. Drain and add to the curry, along with the remaining ¼ teaspoon salt. Stir well to combine.

Serve the curry garnished with the reserved coriander leaves, and lime wedges on the side.

Nutritional analysis per serving: Calories: 380, Fat: 26 g, Saturated Fat: 19 g, Cholesterol: 0 mg, Fiber: 9 g, Protein: 19 g, Carbohydrates: 26 g, Sodium: 440 mg

Seafood

Pacific Coast Bouillabaisse

A bouquet garni consists of a variety of herb sprigs bundled together with some kitchen string. It is used to flavor broths, soups, and sauces. The bouquet is removed prior to serving.

Serves: 6
Prep Time: 30 minutes
Cook Time: 50 minutes

- 450 g firm, lean fish fillets (such as cod, halibut, or bass), cut into 5-cm chunks
- 120 ml extra-virgin olive oil, plus more for drizzling
- sea salt and freshly ground black pepper
- 12 clams, scrubbed
- 2 small onions, chopped
- 2 leeks, chopped, white parts only
- 4 garlic cloves, crushed
- 2 (400-g) cans chopped tomatoes
- 1 tablespoon tomato puree
- 1 liter vegetable stock
- 1 bouquet garni (4 parsley sprigs, 1 bay leaf, 1 thyme sprig, 1 strip orange peel, all tied together with kitchen string)
- pinch of saffron
- 450 g scallops or tender, mild fish fillets (such as snapper or sole) cut into 5-cm chunks
- juice of 1 lime
- chopped fresh tarragon, for garnish

Coat the firm fish chunks with a light drizzle of olive oil and season with a pinch each of salt and black pepper. Cover and chill until ready to use.

Put the clams in a medium saucepan, add 250 ml water, cover, and heat over medium-high heat just until all of the shells have opened, about 3 minutes. Remove the pan from the heat and set aside, covered.

In a large, nonreactive saucepan, heat the 120 ml oil over medium-low heat until shimmering. Add the onions and leeks with a pinch of salt, and cook until softened but not browned, 8 to 10 minutes. Add the garlic and cook until fragrant, 30 seconds to 1 minute. Add the tomatoes with their juices, tomato puree, vegetable stock, bouquet garni, saffron, and another pinch each of salt and black pepper. Simmer for 20 minutes, then remove and discard the bouquet garni.

Transfer the clams to a bowl and strain their cooking liquid through a fine-mesh sieve to remove any sand particles. Add the strained liquid to the soup. Raise the heat to medium-high and bring the soup to a rapid boil. Gently stir in the firm fish, cover, and let cook for 3 to 4 minutes. Add the scallops or tender fish and cook until just opaque, about 3 minutes. Add the clams and bring back to a simmer for 5 minutes, then turn off the heat (be sure to discard any unopened clams).

Add lime juice to taste. Ladle into soup bowls, garnish with fresh tarragon, and serve.

Nutritional analysis per serving: *Calories: 390, Fat: 22 g, Saturated Fat: 3.5 g, Cholesterol: 70 mg, Fiber: 3 g, Protein: 36 g, Carbohydrates: 14 g, Sodium: 390 mg*

CIOPPINO

Cioppino is a seafood stew with its roots in the fishing community of San Francisco. This version uses plaice, squid, and prawns, but you can also add mussels or small clams in their shells, crabmeat, or even lobster. Cooking times for fish and shellfish vary, so always add the heartier shellfish to the pan first—allowing their shells to open if using clams or mussels or for their flesh to turn opaque for crabs and lobsters—then follow with prawns and squid and, finally, the most delicate fish fillets.

Serves: 6
Prep Time: 20 minutes
Cook Time: 30 minutes

- 4 tablespoons extra-virgin olive oil
- 1 teaspoon fennel seeds
- ½ teaspoon dried oregano
- ¼ teaspoon crushed chili flakes, or to taste
- 1 onion, thinly sliced
- 1 small leek, white and light green sections halved lengthwise and thinly sliced
- 2 garlic cloves, thinly sliced
- 1 fennel bulb, thinly sliced
- 1 tablespoon tomato puree
- 2 (400-g) cans chopped tomatoes
- 1 (250-ml) bottle clam juice
- sea salt and freshly ground black pepper
- 450 g medium raw prawns, peeled and deveined
- 450 g plaice or other white fish fillet, cut into 5-cm pieces
- 225 g squid, bodies sliced into thin rings and tentacles halved lengthwise
- chopped fresh basil, for garnish

Warm the olive oil in a large sauté pan or cast-iron casserole over low heat. Add the fennel seeds, oregano, and chili flakes and cook until fragrant, about 2 minutes. Be careful not to burn the spices.

Raise the heat to medium-low and add the onion, leek, garlic, and fennel. Sauté until the vegetables are very soft and just beginning to brown, 7 to 10 minutes.

Add the tomato puree and sauté for 30 seconds, then add the chopped tomatoes with their juices (if you prefer a thicker stew, drain the juices) and the clam juice. Bring to a simmer, then lower the heat and cook for 15 minutes, stirring occasionally. Season with ½ teaspoon salt and a pinch of black pepper.

Add the prawns to the soup and cook just until they begin to turn pink and curl, about 2 minutes. Add the plaice and squid and cook gently, just until they turn white and opaque, about 3 minutes.

Ladle the cioppino into bowls, garnish with basil, and serve.

Nutritional analysis per serving: Calories: 250, Fat: 12 g, Saturated Fat: 2 g, Cholesterol: 170 mg, Fiber: 2 g, Protein: 27 g, Carbohydrates: 13 g, Sodium: 500 mg

MONKFISH TAGINE

Tagine refers to both a clay pot used to cook stews in and the stew itself. The pots are very earthy and calming—much like the food they are used to cook. Tagines typically have warming spices and complex flavors from herbs, spices, and vegetables. But you don't need a clay pot to cook this dish; you'll get the same delicious, comforting results without it.

Serves: 4
Prep Time: 15 minutes
Cook Time: 35 minutes

- 1½ teaspoons coconut oil
- 2 medium onions, halved and sliced
- 1 medium fennel bulb, halved and sliced
- 1 teaspoon grated fresh root ginger
- 1 teaspoon ground cumin
- ½ teaspoon ground cinnamon
- ½ teaspoon ground coriander
- ½ teaspoon sweet paprika
- sea salt and freshly ground black pepper
- 300 ml low-sodium chicken stock
- 1 (225-g) can chopped tomatoes, sieved
- 1 small cauliflower, cored and cut into 5-cm florets
- 450 g cherry tomatoes, halved
- 50 g Kalamata olives, halved
- 4 (175- to 225-g) monkfish fillets
- 2 tablespoons chopped fresh parsley

In a large sauté pan, heat the coconut oil over medium–high heat until shimmering. Add the onions and fennel and sauté until softened, about 10 minutes.

Stir in the ginger, cumin, cinnamon, coriander, paprika, ¼ teaspoon salt, and a pinch of black pepper. Add the chicken stock, sieved tomatoes, and cauliflower and stir well. Reduce the heat to medium–low and let the mixture simmer, stirring occasionally, until the cauliflower is somewhat softened, about 10 minutes.

Stir in the cherry tomatoes and olives. Season the monkfish with a pinch of salt and ¼ teaspoon black pepper. Using a wooden spoon, make four little vegetable "nests" and lay a monkfish fillet in each. Cover the pan and let the fish simmer until it is fully cooked and tender, 12 to 15 minutes.

Serve, garnished with parsley.

Nutritional analysis per serving: Calories: 300, Fat: 9 g, Saturated Fat: 2 g, Cholesterol: 45 mg, Fiber: 8 g, Protein: 31 g, Carbohydrates: 25 g, Sodium: 530 g

THAI GREEN CURRY WITH SOFT-SHELL CRABS

A favorite culinary trick is dredging or coating your meat in flour and egg to create a crisp, delicious crust. This recipe uses coconut flour instead of white flour, which is high-glycemic and inflammatory.

Serves: 4
Prep Time: 20 minutes
Cook Time: 40 minutes

- 1 tablespoon extra-virgin olive oil
- 450 g carrots, peeled and cut into 2.5-cm pieces
- 2 heads baby pak choi, stems cut into 2.5-cm pieces, leaves reserved
- 1 onion, chopped
- 4 tablespoons Thai Green Curry Paste (page 302)
- 1 (400-ml) can full-fat unsweetened coconut milk
- 3 large omega-3 egg whites
- 175 g coconut flour
- ¼ teaspoon sea salt
- 8 soft-shell crabs, cleaned
- 120 ml grapeseed oil
- 150 g baby spinach
- grated zest and juice of 2 limes

Preheat the oven to 120°C/Gas ½.

In a 5-liter cast-iron casserole, heat the olive oil over medium heat until shimmering. Add the carrots, pak choi stems, and onion. Cook until the onion is translucent, 7 to 10 minutes. Add the curry paste and cook, stirring, until fragrant and blended with the vegetables, about 1 minute.

Add the coconut milk and 750 ml water, bring to the boil, and then reduce the heat to a simmer. Cook until the carrots are crisp-tender, 8 to 10 minutes. Cover the casserole and transfer it to the bottom shelf of the oven to keep warm.

Line two baking sheets with a few layers of kitchen paper.

Whisk the egg whites until soft peaks form; transfer to a shallow bowl.

Fill another shallow bowl with coconut flour and the sea salt. Dip one crab into the egg whites, allowing the excess to drip off. Then dip it into the coconut flour, gently patting it to adhere. Carefully place the crab on one of the lined baking sheets. Repeat with the remaining crabs.

In a large cast-iron frying pan, warm the grapeseed oil over medium heat until shimmering, 5 to 7 minutes. The end of a crab leg dipped in the oil will bubble when the oil is ready.

Depending on the size of your pan, gently place 1 or 2 crabs, shell-side down, in the oil. Cook until the shell is pink and the batter has browned, 2 to 3 minutes. Using a thin metal spatula, gently turn the crabs and continue to cook until brown on the bottom, another 1 to 2 minutes. Transfer to the second lined baking sheet and place in the warm oven. Repeat with the remaining crabs.

Remove the casserole from the oven and stir in the spinach and pak choi leaves. Add the lime zest and juice and stir to combine. Divide the curry among four plates and top each with 2 crabs. Serve.

***Nutritional analysis per serving:** Calories: 425, Fat: 28 g, Saturated Fat: 21 g, Cholesterol: 74 mg, Fiber: 12 g, Protein: 15 g, Carbohydrates: 36 g, Sodium: 588 mg*

TANDOORI PRAWNS WITH INDIAN-SPICED CABBAGE

Mustard seeds offer a pungent flavor that can be used to enhance curries and stir-fries. The seeds come from the mustard plant, which is from the same family of plants as cruciferous vegetables such as broccoli and cauliflower. Mustard seeds are acclaimed for their health benefits, ranging from reducing high blood pressure and menopausal symptoms to preventing cancer and calming autoimmune disease. You can find mustard seeds in the spice aisle or Asian section of your supermarket, and you can also order them online.

Serves: 4
Prep Time: 15 minutes, plus marinating time
Cook Time: 20 minutes

- 2 teaspoons sweet paprika
- 1 teaspoon ground ginger
- 1 teaspoon ground cumin
- 1 teaspoon ground coriander
- 1 teaspoon ground turmeric
- 1 teaspoon mild chili powder
- 1¼ teaspoons sea salt
- ¼ teaspoon cayenne pepper
- 120 ml full-fat unsweetened coconut milk
- 2 tablespoons fresh lime juice
- 675 g raw king prawns, peeled and deveined
- 4 to 5 tablespoons grapeseed or coconut oil
- ½ teaspoon yellow or brown mustard seeds
- ½ teaspoon fennel seeds
- 1 red onion, thinly sliced
- 1 tablespoon grated fresh root ginger
- 1 tablespoon finely chopped garlic
- ½ head cabbage (any kind), shredded
- 1 spring onion, thinly sliced
- 4 tablespoons chopped fresh coriander, for garnish
- lime wedges, for serving

Create the Tandoori spice mix by combining the paprika, ground ginger, cumin, coriander, turmeric, chili powder, 1 teaspoon salt, and the cayenne pepper in a small bowl.

In a medium bowl, combine the coconut milk, lime juice, and 2 tablespoons of the Tandoori spice mix and mix well. (The leftover spice mix can be stored in an airtight container.) Add the prawns and toss to coat. Marinate at room temperature for 30 minutes or in the refrigerator, covered, for up to 8 hours.

When you are ready to cook, heat 2 tablespoons of the oil in a large sauté pan over medium heat until shimmering. Add the mustard and fennel seeds and cook just until the mustard seeds start to pop, about 1 minute. Add the onion, grated ginger, and garlic to the pan and sauté until soft and fragrant, about 2 minutes.

Add the cabbage and remaining ¼ teaspoon salt to the pan, turn the heat to high, and sauté the cabbage until it becomes soft and begins to brown, about 10 minutes. You may need to add another tablespoon of oil if the pan seems too dry. (As the cabbage cooks, you can add a few tablespoons of water as needed to release any ingredients that stick to the bottom of the pan.) Transfer the cabbage mixture to a serving platter and stir in the spring onion.

Wash and dry the sauté pan and return it to the stove over high heat. Add the remaining 2 tablespoons oil and heat until shimmering. Drain the prawns from the marinade and reserve any remaining marinade. Using tongs, add the prawns to the hot oil a few at a time. Sauté the prawns quickly, just until they turn pink and begin to curl, 4 to 5 minutes. You may have to work in batches to avoid overcrowding the pan. As the prawns are cooked, place them on top of the cabbage.

Once all of the prawns are cooked, pour any remaining marinade into the pan and cook for 30 seconds, stirring. Pour the cooked marinade over the prawns and cabbage. Garnish with the coriander and serve with lime wedges.

Nutritional analysis per serving: Calories: 315, Fat: 16 g, Saturated Fat: 2 g, Cholesterol: 274 mg, Fiber: 3 g, Protein: 36 g, Carbohydrates: 8 g, Sodium: 563 mg

PRAWN AND THREE-MUSHROOM SAUTÉ WITH CHIVES

A fast yet satisfying lunch or dinner.

Serves: 4
Prep Time: 20 minutes
Cook Time: 15 minutes

- 1½ tablespoons coconut oil
- 675 g medium raw prawns, peeled and deveined
- sea salt and freshly ground black pepper
- 4 medium portobello mushroom caps, cut into 2.5-cm slices
- 200 g oyster mushrooms, sliced
- 40 g shiitake mushroom caps, sliced
- 150 g baby spinach
- 115 g mangetout
- 1 large bunch chives, cut into 5-cm pieces
- 1½ teaspoons grated fresh root ginger
- 1½ teaspoons coconut aminos

In a wok or large nonstick sauté pan, heat ½ tablespoon of the oil over high heat until shimmering. Add the prawns, ¼ teaspoon salt, and a pinch of black pepper and, stirring constantly, sauté until fully cooked, 4 to 5 minutes. Transfer the prawns to a large bowl.

Add another ½ tablespoon of the oil to the pan and reduce the heat to medium–high. Add the portobello slices and sauté, stirring frequently, until just softened, 4 to 5 minutes. Add the oyster and shiitake mushrooms and cook until softened, 2 to 3 minutes. Add to the bowl.

Raise the heat to high and add the remaining ½ tablespoon oil. Add the spinach and mangetout, sautéing until the spinach is wilted, 1 to 2 minutes. Stir in the chives, ginger, and coconut aminos and cook until the chives are wilted, about 1 minute. Transfer the vegetable mixture to the bowl with the prawns and mushrooms, stir to combine, and serve.

Nutritional analysis per serving: *Calories: 250, Fat: 7 g, Saturated Fat: 4.5 g, Cholesterol: 275 mg, Fiber: 4 g, Protein: 39 g, Carbohydrates: 11 g, Sodium: 430 mg*

Fried "Rice" with Prawns

This recipe is a fun alternative to classic fried rice. By replacing the traditional rice with cauliflower, you gain lots of healthy benefits — try it!

Serves: 4
Prep Time: 30 minutes
Cook Time: 15 minutes

- 1 medium cauliflower
- 2 teaspoons grapeseed oil
- 2 red peppers, seeded and sliced
- 225 g mangetout
- 1 (150-g) can water chestnuts, drained
- 75 g raw cashews
- 3 large omega-3 eggs
- 200 g mung bean sprouts
- 450 g large raw prawns, peeled and deveined
- 1 tablespoon toasted sesame oil
- 3 spring onions, chopped, green and white parts separated
- 2 teaspoons finely chopped garlic
- 2 teaspoons grated fresh root ginger
- 1 teaspoon gluten-free, low-sodium tamari
- ¼ teaspoon freshly ground black pepper

Cut the cauliflower in half. Place a box grater over a large bowl and grate each cauliflower half over the big holes of the grater — hold the stem of the cauliflower as you grate.

In a wok or a large sauté pan, heat 1 teaspoon of the grapeseed oil over high heat until shimmering. Cook the red peppers for 1 minute; then, add the mangetout, water chestnuts, and cashews and cook until the vegetables are mostly tender, about 4 minutes.

Meanwhile, in a small bowl, whisk the eggs with 1 tablespoon of water. When the vegetables are tender, push them to the side of the pan. Add the eggs, stirring until scrambled, about 1 minute. Stir in the bean sprouts. Transfer the vegetable mixture to a large serving bowl.

Add the remaining 1 teaspoon grapeseed oil to the pan. Add the prawns and sauté until they are pink and fully cooked, 4 to 5 minutes. Transfer the prawns to the bowl with the vegetables.

Add the sesame oil to the pan and cook the spring onion whites, garlic, and ginger for just 30 seconds. Stir in the grated cauliflower, along with the tamari and black pepper. Cook until the cauliflower is tender, about 3 minutes. Transfer the cauliflower to the bowl with the vegetables and prawns. Garnish with the spring onion greens and serve.

Nutritional analysis per serving: *Calories: 440, Fat: 19 g, Saturated Fat: 3.5 g, Cholesterol: 280 mg, Fiber: 12 g, Protein: 34 g, Carbohydrates: 39 g, Sodium: 525 mg*

HOT AND SPICY PRAWNS WITH CORIANDER

For a less spicy version of this recipe, try using only one jalapeño. And remember that most of a chili pepper's heat is contained in the seeds!

Serves: 4
Prep Time: 15 minutes
Cook Time: 10 minutes

- 3 tablespoons grapeseed oil
- 450 g medium raw prawns, peeled and deveined
- ½ teaspoon ground coriander
- ¼ teaspoon cayenne pepper
- sea salt
- 2 long red sweet chilies (such as Anaheim), seeded and thinly sliced
- 3 jalapeño chilies, seeded and thinly sliced
- 3 leeks, halved lengthwise and cut crosswise into 2.5-cm-thick slices, white and pale green parts only
- 4 garlic cloves, thinly sliced
- 1 bunch coriander, stems included, finely chopped, plus additional leaves for garnish

Heat 1 tablespoon of the oil in a large frying pan over medium-high heat until shimmering. Sprinkle the prawns with the coriander, cayenne, and ¼ teaspoon salt. Add to the hot oil and cook, stirring, until lightly browned and just opaque, 2 to 3 minutes. Transfer to a plate.

Heat another tablespoon of oil in the same pan. Add the sweet chilies, jalapeños, and ¼ teaspoon salt. Cook, stirring occasionally, until crisp-tender, 1 to 2 minutes. Transfer to the plate with the prawns.

Heat the remaining tablespoon of oil in the same pan. Add the leeks, garlic, and a pinch of salt. Cook, stirring occasionally, until the leeks are lightly browned and crisp-tender, about 3 minutes. Add the shrimp, chilies, and chopped coriander and mix well.

Serve garnished with coriander leaves.

Nutritional analysis per serving: *Calories 293, Fat 12 g, Saturated Fat 1 g, Cholesterol 183 mg, Fiber 4 g, Protein 26 g, Carbohydrates 23 g, Sodium 477 mg*

GRILLED SALMON WITH ALMOND-DILL SAUCE

When purchasing salmon, try to choose only wild-caught; it is less environmentally damaging than farmed salmon and much higher in healthy omega-3 fats. If you leave the skin on, you'll get even more of those healthy fats, as they are richest in the skin and just beneath it.

Serves: 4
Prep Time: 10 minutes, plus chilling time
Cook Time: 50 minutes

- 350 ml unsweetened almond milk
- grated zest and juice of 1 lemon
- 3 garlic cloves, crushed
- ½ teaspoon Dijon mustard
- pinch of ground cumin
- freshly ground black pepper
- 3 tablespoons finely chopped fresh dill, plus more for garnish
- 2 tablespoons Mayonnaise (page 299) or Vegenaise
- 2 tablespoons extra-virgin olive oil
- ¼ teaspoon dried sage
- 4 (225-g) boneless, skin-on wild salmon steaks
- ¼ teaspoon sea salt

Combine the almond milk, lemon zest, 1 tablespoon of the crushed garlic, the mustard, cumin, and a pinch of black pepper in a 2-liter saucepan. Bring to the boil over medium heat and cook, stirring occasionally, until the liquid has reduced to about 75 ml, 35 to 40 minutes. Transfer the liquid to a heatproof bowl and chill in the freezer until cool, about 20 minutes (stirring after 10 minutes). Once fully chilled, whisk in the lemon juice, dill, and mayonnaise. Cover and refrigerate until serving time.

Preheat the grill. Line a rimmed baking sheet with foil.

In a small bowl, stir together 1 tablespoon of the oil, the remaining garlic, and the sage. Set aside.

Brush the salmon steaks on both sides with the remaining 1 tablespoon oil and sprinkle with the salt. Place the steaks, skin-side up, on the lined baking sheet. Cook about 12 cm below the grill until the outside is opaque and the skin is beginning to crisp, 4 to 6 minutes. Turn the steaks and continue to cook for another 4 minutes, then brush with the garlic mixture. Continue to cook until the salmon is still pink in the center but warm throughout, about 1 minute. Place the salmon steaks on serving plates, spoon the chilled almond-dill sauce over them, garnish with additional dill, and serve.

Nutritional analysis per serving: *Calories: 454, Fat: 28 g, Saturated Fat: 4 g, Cholesterol: 127 mg, Fiber: 1 g, Protein: 46 g, Carbohydrates: 2 g, Sodium: 358 mg*

ROASTED SALMON WITH GREEN BEANS

We all need a simple "go to" salmon recipe that never lets us down, and this is it!

Serves: 4
Prep Time: 10 minutes
Cook Time: 10 minutes

- 2 tablespoons plus ¼ teaspoon sea salt
- 675 g green beans, trimmed
- 1 teaspoon extra-virgin olive oil
- grated zest of 1 lemon
- 4 (175-g) boneless, skinless wild salmon fillets
- 3 tablespoons Dijon mustard
- 25 g fresh dill, finely chopped
- 1 tablespoon grapeseed oil

Preheat the grill. Line a rimmed baking sheet with foil.

Bring a 5-liter saucepan of water to the boil over high heat. Add 2 tablespoons of the salt. Cook the green beans until crisp-tender, 3 to 4 minutes. Drain the beans in a colander and rinse with cold water. Gently pat the beans dry with kitchen paper and transfer to a large bowl. Toss with the olive oil, lemon zest, and remaining ¼ teaspoon salt. Set aside.

Pat the salmon fillets dry with kitchen paper and place on the lined baking sheet. Spread an equal amount of mustard over the top of each fillet. Divide the dill among the fillets, patting it gently into the mustard. Drizzle the tops of the fillets with the grapeseed oil to prevent the herbs from browning too much.

Place the salmon under the grill and cook until the dill is a bit frizzled and the center of the fish is tender and pink, 6 to 8 minutes. Serve with the green beans on the side.

Nutritional analysis per serving: *Calories: 335, Fat: 16 g, Saturated Fat: 2 g, Cholesterol: 94 mg, Fiber: 5 g, Protein: 37 g, Carbohydrates: 12 g, Sodium: 348 mg*

SALMON BURGERS WITH PICKLED RADISHES AND AVOCADO

I love the zesty zing the pickled radishes provide in this recipe. Enjoy their flavor while your body is flooded with cancer-fighting isothiocyanates and antioxidants like vitamin C.

Serves: 4
Prep Time: 30 minutes
Cook Time: 6 minutes

- 4 or 5 large red radishes, very thinly sliced
- 2 teaspoons fresh lemon or lime juice
- sea salt and freshly ground black pepper
- 450 g boneless, skinless wild salmon fillets, cut into 5-cm pieces
- ¼ red onion, finely diced
- 4 tablespoons chopped fresh mixed herbs (such as parsley, mint, coriander, and/or dill)
- ½ teaspoon grated fresh root ginger
- ½ teaspoon ground turmeric
- ½ teaspoon ground cumin
- ½ teaspoon ground coriander
- 4 tablespoons sesame seeds, preferably mixed black and white
- 1 tablespoon extra-virgin olive oil
- 4 large lettuce leaves (such as romaine, green leaf, or red leaf)
- 1 avocado, stoned, peeled, and sliced, for garnish

In a small bowl, toss the radishes with 1 teaspoon of the citrus juice and ½ teaspoon salt. Set aside.

Place the salmon pieces in a food processor and pulse about 8 times to coarsely chop. Don't let the machine run and puree the fish; you want chickpea-size pieces.

Transfer the chopped fish to a bowl and fold in the onion and herbs. Add the remaining 1 teaspoon citrus juice and ½ teaspoon salt, along with the ginger, turmeric, cumin, coriander, and a pinch of black pepper and mix well.

Spread the sesame seeds on a small plate. Wet your hands, and form the salmon into 4 equal-size patties. Press the sesame seeds onto both sides of each patty and set them on a plate.

Heat the olive oil in a large cast-iron frying pan or sauté pan over high heat until shimmering. Gently place the salmon burgers in the pan and cook until browned on the outside and cooked through, about 3 minutes per side.

Place one lettuce leaf on each plate and place a burger on top. Garnish the burgers with the pickled radishes and sliced avocado and serve.

Nutritional analysis per serving: *Calories: 320, Fat: 21 g, Saturated Fat: 2.5 g, Cholesterol: 60 mg, Fiber: 5 g, Protein: 25 g, Carbohydrates: 7 g, Sodium: 550 mg*

Roasted Salmon and Asparagus with Herb-Avocado Mash

On busy evenings, I love a recipe that simplifies the cooking process, and this recipe does just that—the asparagus and salmon roast at the same time! Dinner is on the table in a jiffy.

Serves: 4
Prep Time: 10 minutes
Cook Time: 10 minutes

- 1 tablespoon grapeseed oil
- 4 (175-g) boneless, skin-on wild salmon fillets
- 24 asparagus spears, trimmed
- 1 tablespoon extra-virgin olive oil
- sea salt and freshly ground black pepper
- 1 avocado, stoned, peeled, and mashed
- 1 tablespoon finely chopped fresh chives
- 1 tablespoon chopped fresh mint
- 1 tablespoon chopped fresh basil
- 1 tablespoon chopped fresh coriander or parsley
- 1 spring onion, finely chopped
- ½ teaspoon fresh lemon or lime juice

Preheat the oven to 200°C/Gas 6.

Brush two rimmed baking sheets with the grapeseed oil. Place the salmon fillets on one sheet and the asparagus on the other sheet. Drizzle the olive oil over the salmon and asparagus, making sure to coat both well. Sprinkle both with ½ teaspoon each salt and black pepper.

Place both baking sheets in the oven and roast until the salmon is just cooked through and the asparagus just begins to wrinkle, 8 to 10 minutes. Depending on the thickness of the asparagus, you may need to leave it in for a few more minutes. Remove both from the oven and set aside.

In a small bowl combine the avocado with the herbs, spring onion, citrus juice, and a pinch of black pepper. Mix well.

Place a salmon fillet on each plate, along with a spoonful of the mashed avocado and 6 asparagus spears. Serve.

Nutritional analysis per serving: Calories: 404, Fat: 25 g, Saturated Fat: 4 g, Cholesterol: 94 mg, Fiber: 6 g, Protein: 37 g, Carbohydrates: 9 g, Sodium: 429 mg

Slow-Cooked Salmon with Asian Greens

Ground turmeric gives the rub for this salmon a beautiful color. Food is medicine, and this recipe certainly celebrates that with the anti-inflammatory compound curcumin in the turmeric, not to mention the anti-inflammatory fats in the salmon. This meal has all the right ingredients to transform your health.

Serves: 4
Prep Time: 10 minutes
Cook Time: 20 minutes

- 1 tablespoon extra-virgin olive oil
- 1 teaspoon ground turmeric
- 1 teaspoon ground coriander
- sea salt and freshly ground black pepper
- 4 (150-g) boneless, skin-on wild salmon fillets
- 3 tablespoons grapeseed oil
- 2 shallots, very thinly sliced
- 550 g pak choi, thinly sliced
- 150 g baby spinach
- 1 teaspoon toasted sesame seeds, for garnish (optional)

Preheat the oven to 140°C/Gas 1. Line a rimmed baking sheet with foil.

In a small bowl, combine the olive oil, turmeric, coriander, ½ teaspoon salt, and ¼ teaspoon black pepper. Rub the mixture on the flesh of the salmon fillets (not the skin). Place the fillets, skin-side up, on the lined baking sheet. Bake until just cooked through, about 20 minutes.

Meanwhile, in a large frying pan, heat the grapeseed oil over medium heat until shimmering. Add the shallots and cook, stirring frequently, until crisp and brown, about 5 minutes. Transfer with a slotted spoon to kitchen paper to drain. Sprinkle with a pinch of salt.

Raise the heat to medium-high and add the pak choi, ¼ teaspoon salt, and a pinch of black pepper. Cook, stirring frequently, until bright green and crisp-tender, about 4 minutes. Add the spinach and season with ¼ teaspoon each salt and black pepper. Cook, stirring, until just wilted, about 1 minute. Divide the greens among four serving plates.

Peel off and discard the salmon skins. Place the fillets on top of the greens and garnish with the crisp shallots and sesame seeds, if desired.

Nutritional analysis per serving: Calories: 370, Fat: 23 g, Saturated Fat: 3 g, Cholesterol: 80 mg, Fiber: 4 g, Protein: 32 g, Carbohydrates: 11 g, Sodium: 430 mg

Chipotle Salmon with Rocket Salad

The balsamic vinegar in this recipe lends a subtle sweetness and depth to the smoky-spicy chipotle. The combination of flavors will quickly captivate your taste buds and make this a family favorite.

Serves: 4
Prep Time: 20 minutes
Cook Time: 40 minutes

- 1 large cauliflower, cored and cut into 5-cm florets
- 2 tablespoons extra-virgin olive oil
- sea salt and freshly ground black pepper
- 1 (200-g) can chipotle peppers in adobo sauce, peppers seeded and finely chopped, 2 teaspoons sauce reserved
- 1 tablespoon balsamic vinegar
- 4 (115- to 175-g) boneless, skin-on wild salmon fillets
- 100 g baby rocket
- 4 tablespoons chopped sun-dried tomatoes
- 4 tablespoons chopped Kalamata olives
- 2 tablespoons pine nuts
- 1 tablespoon cider vinegar
- 1½ teaspoons Dijon mustard

Preheat the oven to 230°C/Gas 8.

Place the cauliflower florets on a large rimmed baking sheet. Drizzle with 1 tablespoon of the olive oil and season with ¼ teaspoon salt and a pinch of black pepper. Toss to coat the cauliflower with the oil and seasonings. Roast the cauliflower, stirring once midway, until it is tender and golden, 25 to 30 minutes. Remove from the oven and reduce the temperature to 200°C/Gas 6.

In a small bowl, stir together the chipotle peppers, adobo sauce, and balsamic vinegar. Place the salmon fillets, skin-side down, in a baking dish. Use a spoon or a brush to coat the top of the salmon with the chipotle mixture. Bake until the salmon is cooked through, 12 to 16 minutes, depending on the thickness.

Meanwhile, in a large bowl, combine the roasted cauliflower, rocket, sun-dried tomatoes, olives, and pine nuts. In a small bowl, whisk together the remaining 1 tablespoon olive oil, the cider vinegar, mustard, and a pinch of salt. Drizzle the dressing over the salad, gently tossing to combine. Serve with the salmon.

Nutritional analysis per serving: Calories: 416, Fat: 25 g, Saturated Fat: 3 g, Cholesterol: 65 mg, Fiber: 8 g, Protein: 30 g, Carbohydrates: 22 g, Sodium: 519 mg

Grilled Salmon with Cucumber Salad

I serve this meal for weekend brunch because the dill and caraway remind me of refreshing, uplifting Sunday mornings.

Serves: 4
Prep Time: 15 minutes
Cook Time: 10 minutes

- 4 tablespoons apple cider vinegar
- 1 tablespoon caraway seeds
- 1 tablespoon yellow mustard seeds
- sea salt and freshly ground black pepper
- 2 large cucumbers, thinly sliced
- 4 (175-g) boneless, skin-on wild salmon fillets
- 150 g baby rocket
- 1 head chicory, thinly sliced
- 25 g chopped fresh dill, plus more for garnish
- 1 tablespoon almond or extra-virgin olive oil
- grated zest and juice of 1 lemon

Combine the vinegar, caraway seeds, mustard seeds, ½ teaspoon salt, and a pinch of black pepper in a large bowl. Add the cucumber and stir to coat. Let stand, stirring occasionally, while you prepare the salmon.

Heat a well-seasoned griddle pan or large frying pan over medium heat. Sprinkle the flesh side of the salmon fillets with ¼ teaspoon each salt and black pepper. Place the fillets, skin-side up, in the pan and cook until the flesh releases easily from the bottom, about 5 minutes. Turn and cook until the salmon is just opaque throughout, about 4 more minutes.

While the salmon cooks, toss the rocket, chicory, dill, and almond oil with the cucumber mixture. Divide the salad among four plates. Top each with a salmon fillet and garnish with the lemon zest, lemon juice, and additional dill. Serve.

Nutritional analysis per serving: *Calories: 339, Fat: 16 g, Saturated Fat: 2 g, Cholesterol: 94 mg, Fiber: 3 g, Protein: 37 g, Carbohydrates: 13 g, Sodium: 525 mg*

ASIAN-SPICED SALMON CAKES

These salmon cakes are moist and full of flavor. Double the batch and call some friends over to enjoy together!

Serves: 4
Prep Time: 30 minutes
Cook Time: 5 minutes

- 2 large cucumbers, halved lengthwise and thinly sliced
- 2 medium shallots, 1 thinly sliced, 1 finely chopped
- 3 tablespoons apple cider vinegar
- 1 tablespoon plus 1 teaspoon gluten-free, low-sodium tamari
- ½ teaspoon toasted sesame oil
- sea salt
- 1 head Chinese leaves, cut into 2.5-cm pieces
- 550 g boneless, skinless wild salmon fillets, cut into 2.5-cm pieces
- 75 g mangetout, trimmed and thinly sliced
- 3 tablespoons Mayonnaise (page 299) or Vegenaise
- 1 tablespoon five-spice powder
- 1 tablespoon grapeseed oil

In a medium bowl, toss the cucumber and sliced shallot with 2 tablespoons of the vinegar, 1 teaspoon of the tamari, the sesame oil, and a pinch of salt. Let stand while you prepare the salmon cakes.

Pulse the Chinese leaves in a food processor until very finely chopped. Transfer to a colander and toss with ¼ teaspoon salt; let stand.

Combine the chopped shallot and remaining 1 tablespoon vinegar in a large bowl. Pulse three-quarters of the salmon in the food processor until finely ground. Transfer to the bowl with the shallot. Pulse the remaining salmon until just coarsely chopped. Transfer to the bowl, along with the mangetout, mayonnaise, remaining 1 tablespoon tamari, five-spice powder, and ¼ teaspoon salt. Squeeze as much liquid as possible out of the Chinese leaves with your hands. Add the Chinese leaves to the salmon mixture. Mix well with your hands and shape into 4 equal-size patties.

Heat the grapeseed oil in a large nonstick frying pan over medium-high heat until shimmering. Add the salmon cakes and cook until browned and just cooked through, 2 to 3 minutes per side. Serve with the cucumber salad on the side.

Nutritional analysis per serving: *Calories: 311, Fat: 15 g, Saturated Fat: 2 g, Cholesterol: 80 mg, Fiber: 2 g, Protein: 31 g, Carbohydrates: 12 g, Sodium: 577 mg*

WHOLE SNAPPER STUFFED WITH SPRING ONION AND GINGER

The result of cooking fish whole is sweet and delicate.

Serves: 4
Prep Time: 15 minutes
Cook Time: 40 minutes

- 1 head Chinese leaves, cut into 8-cm pieces
- 5 large spring onions, cut into 5-cm pieces
- 10-cm piece fresh root ginger, peeled and thinly sliced
- 2 tablespoons toasted sesame oil
- 1 teaspoon sea salt
- 1 teaspoon freshly ground black pepper
- 1 (1.1-kg) whole wild red snapper, scaled, gutted, and butterflied
- 3 tablespoons gluten-free, low-sodium tamari

Preheat the oven to 220°C/Gas 7. Tear off a 120-cm length of foil and a 90-cm length of baking paper. Place the foil on a large rimmed baking sheet, then lay the baking paper on top.

In a large bowl, combine the Chinese leaves, two-thirds of the spring onions and ginger, 1 tablespoon of the sesame oil, and ½ teaspoon each of the salt and black pepper. Mix to coat evenly. Spread the mixture in an even layer on the baking paper to form a bed for the fish.

Place the fish on top of the Chinese leaves and sprinkle the outside and cavity with the remaining ½ teaspoon each salt and black pepper. Stuff the remaining spring onions and ginger slices in the cavity of the fish.

Combine the tamari with 4 tablespoons of water and pour over the fish. Bring up the sides of the baking paper and fold it over the fish to encase it, then bring together the foil edges and crimp tightly to seal.

Bake for 40 minutes. Carefully open the packet and drizzle the remaining 1 tablespoon sesame oil over the fish. Serve with the Chinese leaves.

Nutritional analysis per serving: *Calories: 230, Fat: 9 g, Saturated Fat: 1.5 g, Cholesterol: 40 mg, Fiber: 3 g, Protein: 28 g, Carbohydrates: 11 g, Sodium: 540 mg*

STEAMED RED SNAPPER AND VEGETABLES EN PAPILLOTE

En papillote literally means "in paper." This culinary trick produces a light dish yet doesn't skimp on flavor or texture. Cooking in paper allows you to preserve the crisp nature of lightly cooked vegetables while maintaining the firm flesh of the snapper.

Serves: 4
Prep Time: 35 minutes
Cook Time: 18 minutes

- 325 ml chilled unsweetened coconut cream, liquid poured off, solid cream reserved
- 1 celeriac, peeled and finely chopped
- 325 g cauliflower florets, broken into small pieces
- 2 shallots, thinly sliced
- grated zest and juice of 2 limes
- ½ teaspoon curry powder
- ½ teaspoon sea salt
- 4 (115-g) skinless red snapper fillets
- 2 jalapeño chilies, seeded and thinly sliced

Preheat the oven to 200°C/Gas 6. Place two large rimmed baking sheets in the oven to preheat them.

Set aside 2 tablespoons of the coconut cream. In a medium bowl, combine the remaining coconut cream, celeriac, cauliflower, shallots, lime zest and juice, curry powder, and salt. Set aside.

Fold four 40 x 60-cm rectangles of baking paper in half (forming 40 x 30-cm rectangles), cut each into a half-heart shape, and open (check out an online video tutorial if necessary). Divide the celeriac mixture among the paper hearts, forming a bed on one side of each heart. Place a red snapper fillet on top of each bed of celeriac. Brush each fillet with the reserved coconut cream. Top the fillets with the jalapeño slices.

To seal the packets, fold the paper flap over the snapper; make small overlapping folds along the edges to seal.

Using a large spatula, place the packets on the preheated baking sheets. Bake, rotating the baking sheets midway, until the packets have puffed, 15 to 18 minutes; the fish will be cooked through by then. Transfer each packet to a serving plate. Serve immediately, taking care to open the packets slowly to avoid being burned by the steam.

Nutritional analysis per serving: *Calories: 360, Fat: 17 g, Saturated Fat: 14 g, Cholesterol: 40 mg, Fiber: 6 g, Protein: 29 g, Carbohydrates: 28 g, Sodium: 480 mg*

PAK CHOI STIR-FRY WITH BLACK COD

This dish celebrates the buttery flavor that oily fish offer. Look for mackerel, Arctic char, or sea bass if you can't find black cod. Be sure to pick out any pin bones from the cod that the fishmonger may have missed. Serve with a side of Cauliflower "Rice" (page 264).

Serves: 4
Prep Time: 20 minutes
Cook Time: 16 minutes

- 4 tablespoons grapeseed oil
- 4 (115-g) boneless, skin-on black cod (or other oily fish) fillets
- sea salt
- 3 garlic cloves, finely chopped
- 2.5-cm piece fresh root ginger, peeled and finely chopped
- 225 g shiitake mushrooms, stalks removed, caps cut into 5-mm-thick slices
- 4 spring onions, cut diagonally into 2.5-cm pieces
- 1 tablespoon gluten-free, low-sodium tamari
- 1 red pepper, seeded and thinly sliced
- 450 g baby pak choi, trimmed, halved lengthwise if large

Heat a well-seasoned griddle pan or large frying pan over medium–high heat. Rub 1 tablespoon of the oil all over the fish and sprinkle the flesh side with ¼ teaspoon salt. Place the fillets, skin-side up, in the hot pan. Cook until the flesh releases easily from the pan, about 5 minutes. Carefully turn each piece over and cook just until opaque throughout, about 3 minutes. Transfer to a plate.

While the fish cooks, heat 1 tablespoon of the oil in a large frying pan over medium–high heat until shimmering. Add half of the garlic and ginger and cook, stirring, for 5 seconds. Add the mushrooms, spring onions, 1½ tablespoons of water, and a pinch of salt. Cook, stirring occasionally, until the mushrooms are lightly browned and tender, about 5 minutes. Stir in the tamari, then transfer the mixture to a bowl.

Heat the remaining 2 tablespoons oil in the same pan. Add the remaining garlic and ginger and cook, stirring, for 5 seconds. Add the red pepper, pak choi, 1½ tablespoons of water, and ¼ teaspoon salt. Cook, stirring, just until the vegetables are crisp-tender, about 3 minutes. Return the mushroom mixture to the pan and fold gently to mix. Divide among four serving plates and top with the grilled fish. Serve.

Nutritional analysis per serving: Calories: 367, Fat: 28 g, Saturated Fat: 5 g, Cholesterol: 56 mg, Fiber: 4 g, Protein: 19 g, Carbohydrates: 10 g, Sodium: 489 mg

Miso-Marinated Cod with Fresh Basil and Pak Choi

This is a great last-minute dish.

Serves: 4
Prep Time: 20 minutes
Cook Time: 10 minutes

- 2 tablespoons plus ¼ teaspoon sea salt
- 1 large head pak choi (about 675 g), stems and leaves separated and cut into 1-cm-thick pieces
- 1 teaspoon toasted sesame oil
- 4 tablespoons gluten-free, low-sodium white miso
- 3 tablespoons apple cider vinegar
- 4 garlic cloves, crushed
- ¼ teaspoon cayenne pepper
- 4 (175-g) skinless wild-caught cod fillets
- 4 tablespoons chopped fresh basil, for garnish
- 2 teaspoons toasted sesame seeds, for garnish
- ¼ teaspoon crushed chili flakes, for garnish

Preheat the grill. Line a rimmed baking sheet with foil.

Bring a 5-liter saucepan of water to the boil over high heat. Add 2 tablespoons of the salt. Cook the pak choi stems until they start to become translucent, 2 to 3 minutes. Then, add the leaves and continue to cook until the leaves are tender, another 1 to 2 minutes. Drain the pak choi in a colander, gently pat dry with kitchen paper, and transfer to a medium bowl. Toss with the sesame oil and the remaining ¼ teaspoon salt. Set aside.

In a small bowl, whisk together the miso, vinegar, garlic, and cayenne. Pat the fish dry with kitchen paper and place on the lined baking sheet. Spread the miso mixture over the top of each fish fillet. Place the fish under the grill until the top is a bit dry and the fish is cooked through, 6 to 8 minutes. Garnish the fish and serve with pak choi.

Nutritional analysis per serving: *Calories 221, Fat 4 g, Saturated Fat 1 g, Cholesterol 73 mg, Fiber 2 g, Protein 34 g, Carbohydrates 13 g, Sodium 619 mg*

COD CAKES WITH MISO AUBERGINE

This is one dish you won't want to skip — especially if you love the refreshing, zesty flavor of lime that is beautifully infused in each bite of cod. The miso aubergine is sure to impress, with its unforgettable umami, or savory, flavor.

Serves: 4
Prep Time: 20 minutes, plus chilling time
Cook Time: 40 minutes

- 4½ tablespoons extra-virgin olive oil
- 450 g skinless wild-caught cod fillets
- ¼ teaspoon sea salt
- 3 tablespoons gluten-free, low-sodium white miso
- 1 tablespoon rice wine vinegar
- 1 garlic clove, crushed
- 2 small aubergines, cut crosswise into 1-cm slices
- ½ teaspoon sesame seeds (optional)
- 2 large omega-3 eggs
- 2 spring onions, thinly sliced, plus more for garnish
- ½ teaspoon grated fresh lime zest
- 2 tablespoons fresh lime juice
- 120 g coconut flour
- 120 ml Mayonnaise (page 299) or Vegenaise
- 2 teaspoons wasabi paste

Preheat the oven to 200°C/Gas 6.

Brush a rimmed baking sheet with ½ tablespoon of the oil. Place the cod fillets on the sheet; season with a pinch of salt. Roast until cooked through, 6 to 8 minutes. Transfer the fillets to a plate and refrigerate to cool completely, 10 to 15 minutes; if any moisture accumulates after cooling, pat dry with kitchen paper. With a fork, flake the fish into small pieces.

Preheat the grill. Line a large rimmed baking sheet with foil.

In a small bowl, combine the miso, vinegar, and garlic. Set aside.

Brush both sides of the aubergine slices with 2 tablespoons of the oil and arrange them on the lined baking sheet. Place them about 6 cm under the grill and grill until golden brown and beginning to soften, 10 to 12 minutes, flipping the slices halfway through cooking.

Spread the miso mixture evenly over each slice of aubergine. Return to the grill and cook until the miso is bubbling and the aubergine is tender, 8 to 10 minutes. If the miso begins to get too dark, cover the aubergine with foil and continue to cook. Sprinkle with sesame seeds, if desired. Set aside.

In a large bowl, combine the eggs, spring onions, lime zest and juice, and remaining salt. Fold in the fish and 4 tablespoons of the coconut flour. Place the remaining coconut flour on a plate. Form 8 equal-size cakes, using about 4 tablespoons of fish mixture for each. Dredge the cakes in the flour, gently pressing to adhere.

In a small bowl, whisk together the mayonnaise and wasabi paste and set aside.

Warm the remaining 2 tablespoons of oil in a 25-cm frying pan over medium heat until shimmering. Place 4 cakes in the pan and cook until golden brown, 2 to 4 minutes per side. Repeat with the remaining cakes. Serve with the aubergines and wasabi mayo on the side.

Nutritional analysis per serving: *Calories: 522, Fat: 29 g, Saturated Fat: 8 g, Cholesterol: 168 mg, Fiber: 14 g, Protein: 30 g, Carbohydrates: 37 g, Sodium: 624 mg*

Chicken and Turkey

BRAISED CHICKEN WITH ONIONS AND PEPPERS

The sauce from the chicken, vegetables, and herbs will make you return to this recipe time and time again.

Serves: 4
Prep Time: 25 minutes
Cook Time: 1 hour and 15 minutes ·

- 1 tablespoon coconut oil
- 550 g boneless, skinless chicken thighs
- ½ teaspoon sea salt
- ½ teaspoon freshly ground black pepper
- 4 medium onions, halved and thinly sliced
- 2 green peppers, seeded and thinly sliced
- 4 red peppers, seeded and thinly sliced
- 3 garlic cloves, thinly sliced
- 75 ml apple cider vinegar
- 75 ml low-sodium chicken stock
- ½ teaspoon dried thyme
- 175 to 300 g rocket or baby spinach

In a large cast-iron casserole, warm the oil over medium-high heat until shimmering. Season the chicken thighs with ¼ teaspoon each salt and black pepper. Brown the chicken thighs, 4 to 5 minutes on each side. Transfer the chicken to a plate.

Add the onions to the pan and cook, stirring occasionally, until softened, about 10 minutes. Stir in the peppers and cook for another 10 minutes, stirring occasionally. Add the garlic and continue cooking for 1 minute, stirring constantly.

Add the vinegar, chicken stock, thyme, and remaining ¼ teaspoon each salt and black pepper. Stir well, scraping up the brown bits from the bottom of the pan.

Using a wooden spoon, make four little vegetable "nests" and lay a chicken thigh in each. Bring the liquid to the boil, then reduce to a simmer over low heat. Cover and cook until the chicken is tender and cooked through, about 35 minutes. Check occasionally to make sure the liquid is at a simmer.

Use a slotted spoon to transfer the chicken and vegetables to a platter. Bring the remaining liquid to the boil over high heat. Cook until most of the liquid has evaporated and only a few tablespoons of thickened sauce are left, 5 to 10 minutes.

Divide the rocket among four plates. Top with the vegetables and chicken, drizzle sauce over both, and serve.

Nutritional analysis per serving: *Calories: 320, Fat: 10 g, Saturated Fat: 4.5 g, Cholesterol: 135 mg, Fiber: 7 g, Protein: 30 g, Carbohydrates: 27 g, Sodium: 450 mg*

MOROCCAN CHICKEN AND VEGETABLE STEW

This is a vegetable-loaded version of the classic Moroccan stew called a *tagine*. Tagines are usually made with lamb or chicken, with lots of warm spices, ginger, and dried fruit.

Serves: 4
Prep Time: 30 minutes
Cook Time: 1 hour

- 4 tablespoons extra-virgin olive oil
- 2 onions, diced
- 6 garlic cloves, finely chopped
- 1 tablespoon finely chopped fresh ginger
- 1 teaspoon sea salt
- 2 teaspoons ground turmeric
- 2 teaspoons ground cumin
- 2 teaspoons ground coriander
- 2 teaspoons ground ginger
- ½ teaspoon ground cinnamon
- pinch of cayenne pepper
- 4 boneless, skinless chicken thighs, cut into 5-cm pieces
- ½ cauliflower, cored and cut into 5-cm florets
- 8 to 10 button mushrooms, trimmed and quartered
- 1 aubergine, peeled and cut into 2.5-cm dice
- 1 large red pepper, seeded and cut into 2.5-cm pieces
- 1 courgette, sliced into 1-cm-thick rounds
- 500 ml low-sodium chicken or vegetable stock
- 10 cherry tomatoes, halved
- 50 g sliced green olives
- 25 g flaked almonds
- chopped fresh coriander, for garnish

In a cast-iron casserole or heavy saucepan, heat the olive oil over medium-low heat. Add the onions, garlic, and fresh ginger and sauté gently until the onions begin to caramelize, 10 to 15 minutes.

Turn the heat to low, and add ¾ teaspoon of the salt and all of the dried spices. Sauté the spices and onions until fragrant, about 2 minutes.

Sprinkle the chicken with the remaining ¼ teaspoon salt. Turn the heat to medium, add the chicken to the pan, and sauté for 3 minutes, stirring to coat well with the spices.

Add the cauliflower and mushrooms and sauté until they begin to wilt and soften, about 5 minutes.

Add the aubergine, red pepper, and courgette and sauté until they soften, about 5 minutes.

Add the chicken stock and bring to a simmer. It will look as though there isn't enough liquid, but as the vegetables cook down they will release a lot of water.

Simmer the stew gently, stirring occasionally, until all of the vegetables are tender and the liquid is thickened and reduced, 15 to 20 minutes.

Stir in the tomatoes and cook for 1 more minute. Stir in the olives and almonds. Serve garnished with coriander.

Nutritional analysis per serving: Calories: 410, Fat: 23 g, Saturated Fat: 3.5 g, Cholesterol: 80 mg, Fiber: 12 g, Protein: 23 g, Carbohydrates: 32 g, Sodium: 551 mg

BALSAMIC CHICKEN WITH SAUTÉED BRUSSELS SPROUTS

This dish can be made with any combination of chicken—drumsticks, leg–thigh pieces, or bone-in breast halves. Preshredded Brussels sprouts can be purchased in the prepared-vegetable section of some supermarkets. If you can't find them, thinly slice trimmed sprouts, or substitute thinly sliced green cabbage.

Serves: 4
Prep Time: 20 minutes
Cook Time: 35 minutes

- 4 (175-g) bone-in, skin-on chicken thighs
- sea salt and freshly ground black pepper
- 2 tablespoons extra-virgin olive oil
- 1 medium onion, finely diced
- 3 garlic cloves, finely chopped
- 1 medium celery stalk, diced
- ½ fennel bulb, diced
- 1 small carrot, peeled and diced
- 75 g button or chestnut mushrooms, sliced
- 3 tablespoons balsamic vinegar
- 1 bay leaf
- 1 large thyme sprig or ¼ teaspoon dried thyme
- 250 ml low-sodium chicken stock
- 450 g Brussels sprouts, shredded

Pat the chicken dry with kitchen paper and sprinkle with ½ teaspoon salt and a pinch of black pepper. Heat 1 tablespoon of the olive oil in a large sauté pan over medium–high heat until shimmering. When the oil is hot, add the chicken, skin-side down, and sauté until the skin is golden brown, 2 to 3 minutes. Turn the thighs and sauté for another 2 minutes. Remove the chicken from the pan and set aside.

Add the onion, garlic, celery, and fennel and sauté until the vegetables are soft and beginning to brown, 3 to 5 minutes. Add the carrot and mushrooms and continue to sauté until the mushrooms are very soft and wilted, 2 to 3 minutes.

Return the chicken to the pan. Drizzle the balsamic vinegar over the chicken, add the bay leaf and thyme, and then add the chicken stock. Bring to a simmer, then partially cover the pan and turn the heat to low. Simmer for 15 minutes.

Remove the chicken from the pan and keep it warm. Turn the heat up to medium-high and cook until the sauce has thickened and reduced in volume by half, about 5 minutes more. Return the chicken to the pan, spoon the sauce over the chicken, turn off the heat, and cover the pan.

In another sauté pan, heat the remaining 1 tablespoon olive oil over medium heat until shimmering. Add the Brussels sprouts, season with ½ teaspoon salt, and sauté until very soft, wilted, and beginning to brown, about 10 to 12 minutes. Divide the sprouts among four plates. Discard the bay leaf and thyme sprig (if using) and serve the chicken, vegetables, and sauce over the sautéed sprouts.

Nutritional analysis per serving: *Calories: 340, Fat: 15 g, Saturated Fat: 3 g, Cholesterol: 170 mg, Fiber: 4 g, Protein: 38 g, Carbohydrates: 15 g, Sodium: 568 mg*

FORTY-CLOVE BAKED CHICKEN WITH SWISS CHARD

Don't be alarmed by the amount of garlic called for in this classic recipe; the flavor becomes very mellow and sweet after cooking. This dish tastes great with Rocket and Fennel Salad (page 252).

Serves: 6
Prep Time: 20 minutes
Cook Time: 50 minutes

- 2 tablespoons extra-virgin olive oil
- 8 boneless, skinless chicken thighs
- sea salt and freshly ground black pepper
- ½ teaspoon freshly grated nutmeg
- 40 garlic cloves (from about 4 heads), peeled (see Note)
- 120 ml low-sodium chicken stock
- 1 bunch Swiss chard, stems thinly sliced and leaves roughly chopped
- 6 parsley sprigs, plus additional chopped leaves for garnish
- 6 tarragon sprigs, plus additional chopped leaves for garnish

Preheat the oven to 190°C/Gas 5.

Heat 1 tablespoon of the oil in a large cast-iron casserole over medium-high heat. Sprinkle the chicken with 1 teaspoon salt and ¼ teaspoon black pepper. Add the chicken to the casserole and cook until browned on both sides, about 8 minutes total. Transfer to a plate and sprinkle with the nutmeg.

Add the garlic cloves to the casserole. Cook until just golden, about 30 seconds, stirring constantly to avoid burning the garlic. Add the stock and bring to the boil, stirring and scraping up the browned bits. Return the chicken thighs and their accumulated juices to the casserole and nestle them in the garlic. Top with the Swiss chard stems, parsley sprigs, tarragon sprigs, and ¼ teaspoon salt.

Cover and bake until the garlic is tender and emits a sweet aroma and the chicken is cooked through, about 35 minutes.

Discard the parsley and tarragon sprigs. Using tongs, transfer the chicken to a serving platter. Add the Swiss chard leaves, the remaining 1 tablespoon oil, and a pinch each of salt and black pepper to the casserole. Set over medium heat and stir gently until the chard is just wilted and the garlic cloves have melted into a sauce, about 2 minutes. Spoon the garlicky Swiss chard mixture around the chicken and garnish with chopped parsley and tarragon. Serve.

Note: To peel lots of garlic quickly, separate the cloves from the head and put them in a metal mixing bowl. Place another bowl upside-down on top, hold the edges together, and shake vigorously so that the cloves bang against the insides of both bowls. This is a fun activity for kids—and it's much faster and easier than peeling cloves individually.

Nutritional analysis per serving: Calories: 220, Fat: 10 g, Saturated Fat: 2 g, Cholesterol: 110 mg, Fiber: 1 g, Protein: 24 g, Carbohydrates: 9 g, Sodium: 523 mg

GRILLED CHICKEN WITH BASIL PESTO

One of the best-kept secrets among cooks is how to prepare a moist and tasty boneless, skinless chicken breast: Simply stuff it with herbs and aromatics to enhance the flavor of the meat and give your dish personality and flair.

Serves: 6
Prep Time: 15 minutes
Cook Time: 45 minutes

- 4 tablespoons pine nuts
- 2 garlic cloves, halved
- 50 g fresh basil leaves
- 6 tablespoons extra-virgin olive oil
- 2 tablespoons fresh lemon juice
- 1 teaspoon sea salt
- 6 (115-g) boneless, skinless chicken breasts
- 1 aubergine, sliced into 1-cm-thick rounds
- 300 g baby spinach

In a food processor, pulse together the pine nuts, garlic, basil, 2 tablespoons of the olive oil, the lemon juice, and ¼ teaspoon of the salt until just combined. Transfer the pesto to a bowl.

Working with one chicken breast at a time, hold your knife horizontally and cut the breast almost in half through the middle—stop cutting about 1 cm before you reach the other edge to leave a "hinge." Then you can open up the breast like a book. Repeat with the remaining breasts. Sprinkle the chicken all over with ¼ teaspoon of the salt.

Spread the surface of each chicken breast with an equal amount of the basil pesto. Close the chicken breasts back up and brush the outsides with a little oil.

Heat a well-seasoned griddle pan over medium-high heat. Cook the chicken breasts until golden brown on the outside and no longer pink in the center, 5 to 7 minutes on each side. Remove from the heat and, once cool enough to handle, slice the chicken crosswise into strips.

Meanwhile, preheat the grill. Place the aubergine slices on a baking sheet. Brush both sides of the aubergine with the remaining oil and sprinkle with the remaining ½ teaspoon salt. Grill until browned and tender, 10 to 15 minutes on each side.

Place the spinach on a serving platter. Transfer the auergine to the platter, top with the sliced chicken, and serve.

Nutritional analysis per serving: *Calories: 460, Fat: 31 g, Saturated Fat: 4.5 g, Cholesterol: 95 mg, Fiber: 5 g, Protein: 35 g, Carbohydrates: 12 g, Sodium: 520 mg*

CHICKEN WITH OVEN-ROASTED TOMATOES

I love making a sauce that highlights the fresh, bright flavor of vegetables, roasted to bring out their deeper complexities. This recipe celebrates real food for all of its beauty, flavor, and health benefits.

Serves: 4
Prep Time: 15 minutes
Cook Time: 30 minutes

- 1 yellow pepper, seeded and thinly sliced
- 1 orange pepper, seeded and thinly sliced
- 450 g cherry tomatoes, halved
- 1 shallot, finely chopped
- 4 garlic cloves, thinly sliced
- 2 tablespoons extra-virgin olive oil
- sea salt and freshly ground black pepper
- 450 g boneless, skinless chicken breasts, cut into bite-size pieces
- 2 tablespoons fresh lemon juice
- ¾ teaspoon smoked paprika
- 50 g thinly sliced green olives
- 4 tablespoons finely chopped fresh parsley

Preheat the oven to 230°C/Gas 8. Toss the peppers, tomatoes, shallot, and garlic with the olive oil on a rimmed baking sheet. Season with a pinch each of salt and black pepper. Roast until the peppers are just tender and the tomatoes start to collapse, about 20 minutes.

Meanwhile, in a medium bowl, toss the chicken with 1 tablespoon of the lemon juice and the paprika. Season with a pinch each of salt and black pepper. Scatter the chicken on top of the roasted tomato mixture and roast until the chicken is just cooked through, about 10 minutes.

Add the olives, parsley, and remaining 1 tablespoon lemon juice and toss to combine. Season to taste and serve.

Nutritional analysis per serving: *Calories 208, Fat 8 g, Saturated Fat 1 g, Cholesterol 73 mg, Fiber 3 g, Protein 26 g, Carbohydrates 9 g, Sodium 339 mg*

Pan-Roasted Chicken with Wild Mushroom Ragout

One trick to cooking moist chicken breasts is to use bone-in, skin-on breasts. Here, the delicious browned bits left in the pan after sautéing the chicken are used to flavor the accompanying mushroom ragout.

Serves: 4
Prep Time: 20 minutes
Cook Time: 40 minutes

- 4 (175-g) bone-in, skin-on chicken breasts
- sea salt and freshly ground black pepper
- 4 tablespoons extra-virgin olive oil
- 1 large garlic clove, finely chopped
- 450 g mixed mushrooms (such as button, chestnut, shiitake, and/or oyster), trimmed and thinly sliced
- 1 teaspoon fresh lemon juice
- 250 ml low-sodium chicken stock
- 115 g baby rocket or mixed mesclun greens
- 1 tablespoon finely chopped fresh chives or parsley, for garnish

Preheat the oven to 200°C/Gas 6.

Pat the chicken dry with kitchen paper and season with ½ teaspoon salt and a pinch of black pepper. Heat 1 tablespoon of the olive oil in a large oven-proof sauté pan over high heat until shimmering. Add the chicken, skin-side down, and cook until the skin is golden and releases from the pan, 2 to 3 minutes. Turn the chicken over and transfer the pan to the oven. Cook for 15 to 20 minutes, depending on size. The chicken is done when it feels firm to the touch and the internal temperature is 75°C. Transfer the chicken to a small rack set over a plate or baking tray to catch any juices; do not wash out the pan.

Meanwhile, in a large sauté pan, heat 2 tablespoons of the olive oil over medium heat until shimmering. Add the garlic and cook for 30 seconds. Add the mushrooms and ¼ teaspoon salt and cook, stirring occasionally, until the mushrooms are very soft and beginning to brown, 8 to 10 minutes.

Sprinkle ½ teaspoon of the lemon juice over the mushrooms and add the chicken stock. Simmer until the stock reduces by half and the ragout is thickened, 5 to 7 minutes.

Transfer the mushroom ragout to the pan used to cook the chicken. Add the juices that have collected under the chicken and place the pan over low heat. Stir to release the browned chicken bits from the pan into the mushrooms, then remove from the heat.

Cut the chicken off the bone and into slices. Toss the rocket with the remaining 1 tablespoon olive oil and ½ teaspoon lemon juice. Distribute the rocket among four dinner plates and arrange the chicken slices on top. Spoon the mushroom ragout over the chicken and serve, garnished with the fresh herbs.

Nutritional analysis per serving: *Calories: 280, Fat: 18 g, Saturated Fat: 3 g, Cholesterol: 75 mg, Fiber: 1 g, Protein: 28 g, Carbohydrates: 4 g, Sodium: 490 mg*

POACHED CHICKEN WITH COLESLAW, ALMONDS, AND PEPITAS

Celery seeds give that unique flavor in coleslaw that we all love but can't put our finger on. Don't skip this ingredient because it makes the dish.

Serves: 4
Prep Time: 15 minutes
Cook Time: 20 minutes

- 120 ml Mayonnaise (page 299) or Vegenaise
- 1 tablespoon Dijon mustard
- 1 tablespoon apple cider vinegar
- 1 tablespoon fresh lemon juice
- 6 garlic cloves, 3 crushed and 3 halved
- ¼ teaspoon sea salt
- 1 small green cabbage, finely shredded
- 2 medium carrots, peeled and coarsely grated
- 1 small onion, finely diced
- ¼ teaspoon celery seeds
- 4 (175-g) boneless, skinless chicken breasts
- 4 tablespoons flaked almonds
- 4 tablespoons pumpkin seeds (pepitas)

In a small bowl, whisk together the mayonnaise, mustard, vinegar, lemon juice, crushed garlic, and salt.

In a large bowl, combine the cabbage, carrots, onion, and celery seeds. Add the dressing and toss to coat thoroughly. Cover and refrigerate until ready to serve.

Put the chicken and the halved garlic cloves in a large saucepan. Fill it almost to the top with cold water and bring to the boil over medium–high heat. Reduce the heat to a simmer and cook until the chicken is no longer pink in the center, 10 to 12 minutes or until the internal temperature reaches 75°C. Discard the garlic and transfer the chicken to a chopping board.

While the chicken is cooking, toast the almonds and pumpkin seeds in a small frying pan over medium heat, stirring frequently, until they just begin to brown, 2 to 4 minutes.

Slice the chicken; serve with the slaw, and garnish with toasted almonds and pumpkin seeds.

Nutritional analysis per serving: *Calories: 468, Fat: 19 g, Saturated Fat: 3 g, Cholesterol: 116 mg, Fiber: 9 g, Protein: 44 g, Carbohydrates: 30 g, Sodium: 501 mg*

POMEGRANATE CHICKEN

Ras el hanout is a prized Moroccan spice blend that really ties together the Middle Eastern flavors of this dish. It's available at many large supermarkets and specialty shops, or you can try mixing up your own with the recipe on page 300.

Serves: 4
Prep Time: 20 minutes
Cook Time: 5 minutes

- 60 ml fresh lemon juice
- 4 tablespoons tahini
- 1 garlic clove, halved
- sea salt
- 450 g thin-cut boneless, skinless chicken breasts
- grated zest of 1 lemon
- 2 teaspoons ground sumac (or grated zest of another lemon)
- 2 teaspoons Ras el Hanout (page 300)
- 1 head endive or escarole, chopped
- 1 head radicchio, cut in quarters, cored, and thinly sliced
- 75 g pomegranate seeds
- 4 tablespoons chopped toasted walnuts
- chopped fresh parsley, coriander, and/or mint, for garnish

Combine the lemon juice, tahini, garlic, 4 tablespoons of water, and a pinch of salt in a blender. Blend until smooth, 1 to 2 minutes.

Sprinkle the chicken with the lemon zest, sumac, ras el hanout, and ½ teaspoon salt. Heat a well-seasoned griddle pan over medium-high heat. Add the chicken and cook, turning once, until cooked through, 3 to 4 minutes total. Transfer to a chopping board.

Toss the endive, radicchio, and pomegranate seeds with the tahini dressing and divide among four serving plates. Slice the chicken into strips and arrange on top of the salad. Sprinkle with the walnuts and herbs and serve.

Nutritional analysis per serving: *Calories 341, Fat 17 g, Saturated Fat 2 g, Cholesterol 73 mg, Fiber 8 g, Protein 32 g, Carbohydrates 20 g, Sodium 500 mg*

CHICKEN PROVENÇAL WITH COURGETTES AND PEPPERS

The term *Provençal* refers to food prepared in the style of the French region of Provence, where a fresh, whole-foods culinary approach celebrates the region's tomatoes, onions, olives, and garlic. While some people are intimidated by French cooking, even a novice chef will be able to cook this wholesome dish, which tastes as fantastic as it looks.

Serves: 4
Prep Time: 15 minutes
Cook Time: 35 minutes

- 8 bone-in, skinless chicken drumsticks and/or thighs
- sea salt and freshly ground black pepper
- 1 tablespoon extra-virgin olive oil
- 1 large onion, diced
- 1 celery stalk, diced
- 1 small carrot, peeled and diced
- 8 garlic cloves, halved
- 2 teaspoons tomato puree
- 1 bay leaf
- 1 thyme sprig or ½ teaspoon dried thyme
- 1 small courgette, cut into 5-mm-thick rounds
- 1 small red pepper, seeded and cut into 5-mm-thick strips
- 500 ml low-sodium chicken stock
- 2 tablespoons apple cider vinegar
- 2 tablespoons chopped fresh parsley, for garnish
- 2 teaspoons finely chopped fresh oregano, for garnish (optional)

Pat the chicken dry and season with ¼ teaspoon salt and a pinch of black pepper. In a large sauté pan or cast-iron frying pan, heat the olive oil over medium heat until shimmering. Add the chicken and cook until the pieces are browned all over, about 1 minute per side. Transfer the chicken to a plate.

Add the onion, celery, carrot, and garlic to the pan and sauté until the vegetables are soft and golden brown, 5 to 7 minutes. Stir in the tomato puree and cook for 1 minute. Add the bay leaf, thyme, courgette, and red pepper and cook for another 2 minutes.

Return the chicken to the pan. Add the chicken stock, vinegar, and ¼ teaspoon salt and bring to a simmer. Reduce the heat to low, cover the pan, and braise the chicken for 10 minutes.

Transfer the chicken to a plate and set aside. Increase the heat and simmer the sauce and vegetables until the sauce is reduced by half and the vegetables are very tender, about 10 minutes. Discard the bay leaf and thyme sprig (if using). Return the chicken to the pan and coat it with the vegetables and sauce.

Transfer the stew to a serving platter, sprinkle with the parsley and oregano (if desired), and serve.

Nutritional analysis per serving: *Calories: 260, Fat: 10 g, Saturated Fat: 2 g, Cholesterol: 145 mg, Fiber: 2 g, Protein: 30 g, Carbohydrates: 11 g, Sodium: 510 mg*

RATATOUILLE WITH ROASTED CHICKEN

Ratatouille is a summer vegetable stew from the south of France. Traditionally made with aubergines, peppers, courgettes, tomatoes, and basil, it can be served as a side dish or as a delicious base for roasted or grilled meats or fish. It's also wonderful at brunch, topped with poached eggs.

Serves: 8
Prep Time: 30 minutes
Cook Time: 1 hour

- 1 (1.3-kg) whole chicken
- sea salt and freshly ground black pepper
- juice of ½ lemon
- 2 bay leaves
- 2 tablespoons extra-virgin olive oil
- 4 garlic cloves, finely chopped
- 1 small aubergine, cut into 2.5-cm pieces
- 1 small green courgette, cut into 2.5-cm pieces
- 1 small yellow courgette, cut into 2.5-cm pieces
- 1 red, orange, or yellow pepper, seeded and cut into 2.5-cm pieces
- 1 tablespoon tomato puree
- 225 g canned chopped tomatoes or chopped fresh tomatoes with their juices
- 2 tablespoons chopped fresh basil, plus more for garnish

Preheat the oven to 200°C/Gas 6.

Pat the chicken dry with kitchen paper, then place, breast-side up, in a roasting tin or baking dish. Sprinkle the chicken all over with ½ teaspoon salt and a pinch of black pepper, and squeeze the lemon juice all over the chicken. Place the squeezed lemon half and the bay leaves in the chicken cavity. Tie the legs together with kitchen string, brush with oil, and roast the chicken, basting throughout, until an instant-read thermometer inserted in the thickest part of the thigh reads 75°C, 50 to 55 minutes. Remove the chicken from the oven and allow it to rest for 10 minutes.

When the chicken has been in the oven for about 15 minutes, start the ratatouille. Heat the olive oil in a large sauté pan over medium heat until shimmering. Add the garlic and cook for 30 seconds, then add the aubergine and ¼ teaspoon salt. Cook the aubergine until it is very soft and beginning to brown, 10 to 15 minutes. It will stick to the pan a little, thanks to the natural sugars caramelizing. If it begins to burn, loosen the aubergine by stirring gently and adding a teaspoon or two of water if necessary.

When the aubergine is very soft, add the courgettes and pepper and cook until the vegetables are all very soft, about 10 minutes. The pan may still be sticky. If it looks like it's getting too dark, lower the heat.

Add the tomato puree and chopped tomatoes and cook for another 10 minutes, stirring and scraping the pan with a wooden spoon. All of the sticky bits on the bottom should release and be stirred into the ratatouille. Remove the pan from the heat and stir in the basil.

Carve the chicken into 8 pieces and serve over the ratatouille. Garnish with additional basil.

Nutritional analysis per serving: *Calories: 550, Fat: 45 g, Saturated Fat: 8 g, Cholesterol: 125 mg, Fiber: 3 g, Protein: 27 g, Carbohydrates: 8 g, Sodium: 420 mg*

Southwestern Chicken Wraps

Hot chilies are great detoxifiers which gives your metabolism—and your taste buds!—a little kick.

Serves: 4
Prep Time: 15 minutes
Cook Time: 15 minutes

- 4 (175-g) boneless, skinless chicken breasts
- ¾ teaspoon sea salt
- 4 tablespoons Mayonnaise (page 299) or Vegenaise
- ½ red onion, finely chopped
- 3 tablespoons chopped fresh coriander, plus additional coriander sprigs for serving
- grated zest and juice of 3 limes
- 2 jalapeño chilies, seeded and finely chopped
- 2 teaspoons ground cumin
- 1 romaine lettuce heart, separated into leaves
- 1 avocado, stoned, peeled, and thinly sliced
- lime wedges, for serving
- hot chili sauce, for serving (optional)

Put the chicken in a large saucepan. Fill it almost to the top with cold water and add ½ teaspoon of the salt. Bring the water to the boil over medium-high heat. Reduce the heat to a simmer and cook until the chicken is no longer pink in the center, 10 to 12 minutes.

Transfer the chicken to a chopping board. When cool enough to handle, shred the meat with your hands. In a large bowl, combine the shredded chicken, mayonnaise, onion, chopped coriander, lime zest and juice, jalapeños, cumin, and remaining ¼ teaspoon salt. Mix well.

Serve the chicken salad alongside the remaining ingredients. Have your guests wrap the chicken in the lettuce and top with garnishes.

Nutritional analysis per serving: *Calories: 360, Fat: 15 g, Saturated Fat: 3 g, Cholesterol: 112 mg, Fiber: 8 g, Protein: 40 g, Carbohydrates: 18 g, Sodium: 378 mg*

TOMATILLO CHICKEN

This recipe is fun and suitable for little helpers. Have the kids test the tomatillo sauce after blending to make sure it tastes just right. Then, have them wash their hands and help you shred the chicken. Inviting kids to help prepare meals is a great way to convert picky eaters into adventurous diners. If you are unable to get hold of tomatillos, substitute underripe tomatoes with a dash of lime juice.

Serves: 4
Prep Time: 20 minutes
Cook Time: 40 minutes

- 1 medium onion, quartered
- 2 large bone-in, skinless chicken breasts (or 4 [175-g] boneless, skinless chicken breasts if bone-in unavailable)
- ¾ teaspoon sea salt
- 3 large tomatillos, husked and quartered
- 60 g toasted pumpkin seeds, plus more for garnish
- 1 bunch coriander, plus additional chopped leaves for garnish
- 2 serrano chilies, seeded and chopped
- 1 garlic clove, halved
- 150 g baby kale
- 1 tablespoon grapeseed oil

Reserve one-quarter of the onion. Place the remaining onion and the chicken in a large saucepan. Add 1 liter water and ½ teaspoon of the salt and bring to the boil. Reduce the heat to low and poach until the chicken is just cooked through, about 15 minutes. Transfer the chicken to a plate, discard the onion, and reserve the cooking liquid.

Place the tomatillos, pumpkin seeds, coriander, chilies, garlic, reserved onion, half the kale leaves, 250 ml of the chicken cooking liquid, and the remaining ¼ teaspoon salt in a blender. Puree until very smooth, 1 to 2 minutes.

Heat the oil in a large saucepan over medium-low heat. Add the tomatillo mixture; be careful, as it will splatter. Cook, stirring continuously, until thickened to a paste, about 10 minutes. Stir in 350 ml of the chicken cooking liquid. Simmer, stirring occasionally, for 10 more minutes.

Pull the chicken meat from the bones and tear it into large chunks. Add the chicken and remaining kale to the pan and gently stir until the chicken is hot and the kale just wilts, about 1 minute.

Divide among four serving plates, garnish with pumpkin seeds and coriander, and serve.

Nutritional analysis per serving: Calories: 370, Fat: 18 g, Saturated Fat: 3 g, Cholesterol: 85 mg, Fiber: 4 g, Protein: 36 g, Carbohydrates: 16 g, Sodium: 488 mg

Tuscan Chicken Cacciatore

I love inviting people over for dinner, and there is nothing easier than a one-pot meal when you are cooking for company. The next time you have extra friends and family members joining you at the table, simply double this recipe.

Serves: 4
Prep Time: 15 minutes
Cook Time: 1 hour

- 1 tablespoon coconut oil
- 550 g bone-in, skinless chicken thighs
- sea salt and freshly ground black pepper
- 2 medium onions, chopped
- 2 red or green peppers, seeded and chopped
- 2 courgettes, diced
- 300 g button or chestnut mushrooms, trimmed and halved
- 25 g fresh basil leaves, plus 2 tablespoons chopped fresh basil for garnish
- 2 (400-g) cans whole tomatoes
- ½ teaspoon dried thyme
- ½ teaspoon dried oregano

In a large cast-iron casserole, heat the oil over medium-high heat until shimmering. Season the chicken thighs with ¼ teaspoon salt and a pinch of black pepper. Brown the chicken in the hot oil, cooking for 3 to 4 minutes on each side. Transfer the chicken to a plate.

Add the onions and peppers to the pan and cook, stirring occasionally, until softened, about 10 minutes. Stir in the courgettes and mushrooms, and continue cooking for just a few minutes.

Add the basil leaves, stirring until wilted. Add the tomatoes with their juices, thyme, oregano, and ¼ teaspoon each salt and black pepper. Stir to combine, using the back of a wooden spoon to cut the tomatoes in half. Return the chicken to the pan and reduce the heat so the liquid is at a simmer. Cover and cook until the chicken is fully cooked, about 30 minutes.

Transfer the chicken to a plate and tent with foil to keep warm. Bring the vegetables and sauce to the boil over high heat and cook until about half of the liquid has evaporated, 5 to 8 minutes.

Serve the chicken with the vegetables and sauce, garnished with the chopped basil.

Nutritional analysis per serving: *Calories: 320, Fat: 10 g, Saturated Fat: 4.5 g, Cholesterol: 135 mg, Fiber: 5 g, Protein: 33 g, Carbohydrates: 24 g, Sodium: 460 mg*

Yellow Curry with Chicken Meatballs

Adding turmeric to your dishes is a great way to boost your intake of a powerful anti-inflammatory. The luscious curry served over these meatballs is light and refreshing but also creamy and satisfying.

Serves: 4
Prep Time: 30 minutes, plus chilling time
Cook Time: 20 minutes

- 1 large onion, finely chopped
- 5-cm piece fresh root ginger, peeled and finely chopped
- 1 tablespoon plus 1 teaspoon yellow curry powder
- ¾ teaspoon sea salt
- 450 g minced chicken
- 4 lemongrass stalks, roughly chopped
- juice of 2 limes, plus grated zest of 1 lime
- 1 teaspoon ground turmeric
- 500 ml low-sodium chicken stock
- 250 ml full-fat unsweetened coconut milk
- 1 red pepper, seeded and finely chopped
- 1 jalapeño chili, seeded and finely chopped
- 1 bunch coriander (including stems), finely chopped

In a large bowl, combine 2 tablespoons of the onion, 1 tablespoon of the ginger, 1 tablespoon of the curry powder, and ½ teaspoon of the salt. Add the chicken and mix gently with your hands until well combined. Cover the bowl and refrigerate for 15 to 20 minutes.

In a food processor, pulse the lemongrass until very finely chopped, with no bristly strands remaining, scraping the bowl occasionally. Transfer to a large saucepan. Add the remaining ginger and onion, the lime juice and zest, the turmeric, and the remaining 1 teaspoon curry powder. Stir in the chicken stock and coconut milk and bring to the boil over medium-high heat. Reduce the heat to medium to maintain a steady simmer.

Form the chilled chicken mixture into 2.5-cm balls. Carefully drop them into the simmering curry. Adjust the heat to maintain a simmer and simmer until the meatballs are cooked through, about 15 minutes. Season with the remaining ¼ teaspoon salt.

Fold most of the red pepper, jalapeño, and coriander into the curry sauce, reserving a small amount of each for garnish. Simmer until just heated through, about 2 minutes. Divide among four serving bowls, garnish with the reserved pepper, jalapeño, and coriander, and serve.

Nutritional analysis per serving: Calories: 332, Fat: 22 g, Saturated Fat: 13 g, Cholesterol: 98 mg, Fiber: 2 g, Protein: 23 g, Carbohydrates: 13 g, Sodium: 459 mg

RED CURRY STEW WITH CHICKEN AND AUBERGINE

Here is another one-pot meal you will be thankful to have in your meal plan rotation. This hearty stew has just the right amount of heat, but feel free to add a pinch of cayenne if you want even more spice.

Serves: 4
Prep Time: 20 minutes
Cook Time: 45 minutes

- 1 tablespoon coconut oil
- 450 g boneless, skinless chicken thighs
- sea salt and freshly ground black pepper
- ½ medium red onion, sliced
- 1 teaspoon chili powder
- 1 teaspoon grated fresh root ginger
- 1 (400-ml) can full-fat unsweetened coconut milk
- 1 large aubergine, diced
- 1 courgette, diced
- 3 or 4 red bird's eye chilies, seeded and halved lengthwise
- 900 g cherry or baby plum tomatoes
- 225 green beans, trimmed and cut into 5-cm pieces
- 2 spring onions, chopped
- 20 g fresh coriander, chopped
- grated zest of 1 lime
- juice of 2 limes
- 3 tablespoons chopped almonds

In a large sauté pan, heat ½ tablespoon of the coconut oil over medium-high heat until shimmering. Season the chicken thighs with ¼ teaspoon salt and a pinch of black pepper and add them to the pan. Brown the chicken in the hot oil, cooking for 2 to 3 minutes per side. Transfer the chicken to a plate.

Add the remaining ½ tablespoon coconut oil to the sauté pan. Add the onion and sauté until softened, about 5 minutes.

Add the chili powder and ginger and cook, stirring constantly, for just 30 seconds. Add the coconut milk and 175 ml water and stir to combine. Stir in the aubergine, courgette, chilies, and ¼ teaspoon each salt and black pepper. Return the chicken to the pan. Bring the liquid to the boil, cover, and reduce the heat so the stew stays at a simmer. Cook until the chicken is cooked through, about 20 minutes.

Add the tomatoes and green beans and stir to combine. Continue to simmer, uncovered, for 10 minutes.

Remove the pan from the heat. Stir in the spring onions, coriander, and lime zest and juice. Remove the chilies from the dish (if desired), garnish with the almonds, and serve.

Nutritional analysis per serving: Calories: 510, Fat: 33 g, Saturated Fat: 23 g, Cholesterol: 135 mg, Fiber: 9 g, Protein: 30 g, Carbohydrates: 26 g, Sodium: 450 mg

Ginger-Lemon Chicken with Spinach

This is a true chicken dish for the soul. When you are feeling a bit run down and need a nourishing meal to warm you from the inside out, look no further than your kitchen and this recipe to nurture your body, mind, and spirit.

Serves: 4
Prep Time: 20 minutes
Cook Time: 1 hour

- 5-cm piece fresh root ginger, peeled and finely chopped
- sea salt
- 3 tablespoons grapeseed oil
- 1 (1.6 kg) whole chicken
- 2 lemons, 1 sliced into thin rounds, 1 cut into wedges for serving
- 250 g baby spinach
- ¼ teaspoon crushed chili flakes

Preheat the oven to 220°C/Gas 7.

In a small bowl, use a spoon to mash together the ginger, 2 tablespoons salt, and 2 tablespoons of the oil. Set aside.

Pat the chicken dry with kitchen paper. Using your fingers, gently loosen the skin from the chicken breasts. Being careful not to tear the skin, spread half of the ginger-salt paste evenly between the skin and meat; pat the skin back down. Rub the remaining paste inside the chicken cavity. Tuck the entire sliced lemon into the cavity (you may have to cut a few slices in half).

Tie the chicken legs together with cotton kitchen string; tuck the wing tips underneath. Rub the chicken with the remaining 1 tablespoon oil. Place the chicken, breast-side up, in a roasting tin.

Roast the chicken, occasionally basting with the pan juices, until golden-brown, 50 to 55 minutes; an instant-read thermometer inserted in the thickest part of the thigh should read 75°C. Transfer the chicken to a chopping board and tent with foil, reserving the hot roasting tin; allow the chicken to rest for 10 minutes before carving.

Scatter the spinach over the pan juices in the roasting tin. Place the tin back in the oven until the spinach has begun to wilt, 2 to 3 minutes. Toss the spinach in the hot tin until it is fully wilted and dressed with pan juices. Season with a pinch of salt and the chili flakes. Carve the chicken and serve with the spinach and lemon wedges on the side.

Nutritional analysis per serving: *Calories: 480, Fat: 36 g, Saturated Fat: 8 g, Cholesterol: 128 mg, Fiber: 2 g, Protein: 34 g, Carbohydrates: 5 g, Sodium: 460 mg*

Moroccan-Style Chicken

The blend of spices in this dish creates aromatic, authentic Moroccan flavors with no tagine necessary! The lemon loses its acidic tartness in the oven, adding savory depth to the sauce with just a bright zing at the finish. Pair with Green Beans and Almonds (page 254).

Serves: 6
Prep Time: 20 minutes
Cook Time: 40 minutes

- 1 tablespoon fennel seeds
- 1 tablespoon cumin seeds
- 2 teaspoons coriander seeds
- 1 teaspoon ground cinnamon
- 1 teaspoon paprika
- ½ teaspoon Aleppo pepper or ¼ teaspoon crushed chili flakes
- 1 teaspoon sea salt
- 2 tablespoons plus 1 teaspoon extra-virgin olive oil
- 3 small fennel bulbs, each cut into 8 wedges, fronds reserved
- 3 medium shallots, sliced
- 6 (115-g) boneless, skinless chicken thighs
- 1 lemon, very thinly sliced and seeded
- 4 tablespoons finely chopped green olives
- 2 large tomatoes, diced

Preheat the oven to 250°C/Gas highest setting.

In a small frying pan, heat the fennel, cumin, and coriander seeds over medium heat, tossing occasionally, until fragrant and toasted, about 3 minutes. Cool, then transfer to a spice grinder and coarsely grind. Transfer the spices to a large bowl and stir in the cinnamon, paprika, pepper, ¾ teaspoon of the salt, and 2 tablespoons of the oil. Add the fennel wedges, shallots, and chicken and mix until everything is evenly coated.

Spread the chicken and vegetables evenly on a large rimmed baking sheet. Roast until the chicken is cooked through and the vegetables are tender, about 40 minutes.

Meanwhile, toss the lemon slices with the remaining 1 teaspoon oil until well coated. Spread in a single layer on a second baking sheet. Roast alongside the chicken until golden brown and tender, about 30 minutes. Transfer the lemons to a chopping board. When cool enough to handle, chop very finely (including the peel) and transfer to a medium bowl.

Finely chop the reserved fennel fronds. Add half of the chopped fronds to the lemons and mix in the olives, tomatoes, and remaining ¼ teaspoon salt.

Divide the chicken and roasted vegetables among six serving plates and drizzle with the pan juices. Spoon the tomato mixture on top, garnish with the remaining chopped fennel fronds, and serve.

Nutritional analysis per serving: *Calories: 250, Fat: 11 g, Saturated Fat: 2 g, Cholesterol: 110 mg, Fiber: 6 g, Protein: 25 g, Carbohydrates: 15 g, Sodium: 522 mg*

Coconut Curry Chicken Soup with Almonds

Each ingredient in this soup contains immune-boosting nutrients and phytonu-trients that prevent disease. Double the batch and freeze half so that you have soup on hand the next time someone you love is feeling under the weather.

Serves: 4
Prep Time: 15 minutes
Cook Time: 30 minutes

- 1 tablespoon coconut oil
- 3 medium shallots, thinly sliced
- 2 to 3 teaspoons mild curry powder
- ½ teaspoon ground turmeric
- ½ teaspoon ground ginger
- ¼ teaspoon sea salt
- ¼ teaspoon freshly ground black pepper
- 1 liter low-sodium chicken stock
- 450 g thin-cut boneless, skinless chicken breasts
- 1 (400-ml) can full-fat unsweetened coconut milk
- 40 g shiitake mushroom caps, sliced
- 100 g sugar snap peas, sliced
- 1 red pepper, seeded and chopped
- 20 g fresh coriander, chopped
- 2 spring onions, chopped
- juice of 2 limes
- 4 tablespoons flaked almonds
- 1 teaspoon toasted sesame oil

In a medium saucepan, heat the oil over medium-high heat until shim-mering. Add the shallots and sauté until translucent, 3 to 4 minutes.

Stir in 2 teaspoons of the curry powder, the turmeric, ginger, salt, and black pepper and cook for 30 seconds. Pour in the chicken stock and 250 ml water; stir to combine. Bring the liquid to the boil over high heat.

Add the chicken breasts, trying to make sure they are submerged in the liquid. Reduce to a simmer and cook until the chicken is cooked through, 10 to 15 minutes (cut into one of the thicker pieces to verify that it is no longer pink inside). Transfer the chicken to a bowl and let cool.

Add the coconut milk, mushrooms, sugar snap peas, and red pepper to the pan. Let the soup continue to simmer for 7 to 10 minutes. Taste and add more curry powder, if desired.

Meanwhile, cut the chicken into bite-size pieces. Remove the soup from the heat and stir in the chicken, coriander, spring onions, and lime juice. Ladle the soup into four bowls. Garnish with almonds, drizzle with sesame oil, and serve.

Nutritional analysis per serving: *Calories: 480, Fat: 33 g, Saturated Fat: 23 g, Cholesterol: 100 mg, Fiber: 3 g, Protein: 35 g, Carbohydrates: 15 g, Sodium: 351 mg*

SOUTHWESTERN TURKEY CHILI

This chili will flood your body with a healthy dose of potassium, an important blood pressure regulator.

Serves: 8
Prep Time: 20 minutes
Cook Time: 30 minutes

- 1 tablespoon extra-virgin olive oil
- 900 g minced turkey, preferably dark meat
- 1 onion, finely chopped
- 2 peppers (any color), seeded and finely chopped
- 2 jalapeño chilies, seeded and finely chopped
- 6 garlic cloves, finely chopped
- 3 tablespoons mild chili powder
- 1½ tablespoons smoked paprika
- 1½ tablespoons ground cumin
- 1½ tablespoons garlic powder
- sea salt and freshly ground black pepper
- 700 ml passata
- 2 (400-g) cans chopped tomatoes
- 1 avocado, stoned, peeled, and sliced, for garnish
- 2 tablespoons chopped fresh coriander, for garnish
- 1 spring onion, sliced, for garnish

In a large saucepan, heat the oil over medium–high heat until shimmering. Add the turkey and cook, breaking up with a spoon, until no longer pink, 5 to 7 minutes. Stir in the onion, peppers, jalapeños, garlic, chili powder, paprika, cumin, garlic powder, 1 teaspoon salt, and a pinch of black pepper. Add the passata and the canned tomatoes with their juices, reduce the heat to medium, and cook, stirring occasionally, for 20 to 25 minutes. Serve, topped with garnishes.

Nutritional analysis per serving: *Calories: 310, Fat: 16 g, Saturated Fat: 3.5 g, Cholesterol: 85 mg, Fiber: 6 g, Protein: 25 g, Carbohydrates: 21 g, Sodium: 460 mg*

SPICED TURKEY AND COURGETTE MEATBALLS

Minced turkey makes for tasty meatballs, meatloaf, burgers, or chili. Pair with a vegetable side dish such as Mashed Cauliflower with Horseradish (page 265).

Serves: 4
Prep Time: 20 minutes
Cook Time: 15 minutes

- 450 g minced turkey (preferably dark meat)
- 1 small courgette, grated
- 1 shallot, finely chopped
- 1 garlic clove, finely chopped
- 1 large omega-3 egg, beaten
- 1 teaspoon dried oregano
- ¾ teaspoon sea salt
- ½ teaspoon Aleppo pepper or ¼ teaspoon crushed chili flakes
- ½ teaspoon fennel seeds, crushed
- ½ teaspoon dried sage
- 2 tablespoons grapeseed oil, plus more if needed
- chopped fresh basil or chives, for garnish

Preheat the oven to 200°C/Gas 6. In a large bowl, combine all of the ingredients except the grapeseed oil and basil and mix well. Using wet hands, form the mixture into 12 balls, each about the size of a tangerine.

Heat the grapeseed oil in a large oven-proof sauté pan over medium-high heat until shimmering. Place the meatballs in the hot pan, leaving space between them. (Depending on the size of your sauté pan, you may need to cook the meatballs in batches.) Cook, using a large spoon to turn the meatballs gently, until brown, about 30 seconds per side. The meatballs will be soft, so turn carefully.

Transfer the sauté pan to the oven and bake until the meatballs feel firm to the touch, 8 to 10 minutes. Garnish with basil and serve.

Nutritional analysis per serving: *Calories: 262, Fat: 19 g, Saturated Fat: 5 g, Cholesterol: 145 mg, Fiber: 1 g, Protein: 21 g, Carbohydrates: 2 g, Sodium: 520 mg*

CHILI-SPICED TURKEY MEATLOAF WITH ROASTED CARROT SALAD

Protein keeps the nighttime munchies at bay. If you tend to feel hungry or have a habit of grazing after dinner, this meal will help you meet your intake of nutritious protein, which keeps your blood sugar stable and prevents cravings.

Serves: 8
Prep Time: 20 minutes
Cook Time: 1 hour

- 6 garlic cloves, halved
- 2 celery stalks, coarsely chopped
- 1 small onion, coarsely chopped
- 60 g coconut flour
- 3 large omega-3 eggs, beaten
- 3 tablespoons paprika
- 1 tablespoon chili powder
- sea salt
- 900 g minced turkey (preferably dark meat)
- 900 g carrots, peeled and cut into large batons
- 2 tablespoons plus 2 teaspoons grapeseed oil
- 60 g pumpkin seeds
- 20 g fresh coriander, chopped
- ½ teaspoon ground cumin

Preheat the oven to 190°C/Gas 5.

In the bowl of a food processor, pulse the garlic, celery, and onion until very finely chopped. Transfer the vegetables to a large bowl and add the coconut flour, eggs, 1 tablespoon of the paprika, the chili powder, and 1 teaspoon salt. Add the turkey and, using your hands, mix until combined; do not overmix or the meatloaf will be dense.

Gently pat the meat into a loaf and place in a 20-by 12-cm loaf tin. Do not press down or into the corners. Place the tin on a rimmed baking sheet and bake on the top shelf for 50 minutes.

While the meatloaf cooks, toss the carrots with 2 teaspoons of the oil and a pinch of salt on two large rimmed baking sheets. Roast on the bottom and middle shelves of the oven, tossing once halfway through, until tender, 15 to 20 minutes. Remove and tent with foil to keep warm.

When the meatloaf has baked for 50 minutes, stir together the remaining 2 tablespoons paprika and 2 tablespoons grapeseed oil. Brush the top of the loaf with the mixture and continue cooking until an instant-read thermometer inserted into the thickest part of the loaf registers 68°C, about 10 more minutes. Remove from the oven; let rest for 10 minutes before slicing.

While the meatloaf rests, place the pumpkin seeds in a small frying pan and lightly toast them over medium-low heat, stirring frequently, until they take on the slightest hint of color, 3 to 5 minutes.

Combine the carrots, pumpkin seeds, coriander, and cumin, tossing to combine. Serve with the meatloaf.

Nutritional analysis per serving: *Calories: 395, Fat: 23 g, Saturated Fat: 5 g, Cholesterol: 168 mg, Fiber: 8 g, Protein: 29 g, Carbohydrates: 20 g, Sodium: 521 mg*

ROASTED TURKEY WITH HERB PASTE

If you are like me and wish Thanksgiving came around monthly instead of yearly, then you will love this recipe.

Serves: 6
Prep Time: 20 minutes
Cook Time: 1 hour

- 1 (450-g) boneless, skinless turkey breast
- ¼ teaspoon sea salt
- ¼ teaspoon freshly ground black pepper
- 2 spring onions, roughly chopped
- 2 garlic cloves, halved
- 50 g fresh parsley leaves
- leaves from 4 to 6 thyme sprigs
- leaves from 1 large rosemary sprig
- 1 tablespoon Dijon mustard
- 1 tablespoon extra-virgin olive oil
- 1 lemon, sliced into 6 rounds

Preheat the oven to 180°C/Gas 4. Place the turkey breast in a baking dish and season with the salt and black pepper.

In the bowl of a food processor, combine the spring onions, garlic, parsley, thyme, rosemary, mustard, and olive oil. Pulse until a thick paste forms, 30 seconds to 1 minute.

Spread one-half to two-thirds of the herb paste over the top of the turkey breast. Layer the lemon slices over the herb paste.

Roast the turkey until an instant-read thermometer inserted into the thickest part reads 75°C, 45 to 60 minutes. Remove the turkey from the oven, tent with foil, and let rest for 10 to 15 minutes.

Remove the lemon slices and slice the turkey. Arrange the turkey slices on a platter and top with additional herb paste. Serve.

Nutritional analysis per serving: *Calories: 231, Fat: 7 g, Saturated Fat: 1 g, Cholesterol: 60 mg, Fiber: 2 g, Protein: 36 g, Carbohydrates: 3 g, Sodium: 230 mg*

TURKEY BURGERS

For a heartier meal, try pairing these burgers with Onion-Leek Soup (page 126).

Serves: 4
Prep Time: 20 minutes
Cook Time: 15 minutes

- 4 tablespoons apple cider vinegar
- ¾ teaspoon sea salt
- ½ teaspoon freshly ground black pepper
- 350 g radishes, very thinly sliced
- 1 teaspoon fresh lime juice
- 2 tablespoons Mayonnaise (page 299) or Vegenaise
- 450 g minced turkey
- 1 large courgette, coarsely grated
- 1 bunch chives, thinly sliced
- 1 large omega-3 egg, beaten
- 1 teaspoon ancho chili powder
- 1 teaspoon ground cumin
- ¼ teaspoon cayenne pepper
- 2 tablespoons grapeseed oil
- 16 red lettuce leaves
- 2 tomatoes, thinly sliced

Combine the vinegar and ¼ teaspoon each of the salt and black pepper in a medium bowl. Add the radishes, turn to coat, and let stand.

In a small bowl, whisk the lime juice into the mayonnaise; set aside.

Combine the turkey, courgettes, chives (reserve a little for the garnish), egg, chili powder, cumin, cayenne, and remaining ½ teaspoon salt and ¼ teaspoon black pepper in a large bowl. Form into 4 equal-size patties.

Heat the oil in a large nonstick frying pan over medium heat until shimmering. Add the patties and cook, turning once, until cooked through, about 15 minutes.

For each serving, stack 2 lettuce leaves and place 1 burger in the center. Top each burger with some of the lime-mayo mixture, tomato slices, pickled radishes, and reserved chives. Sandwich with 2 more lettuce leaves and serve with any remaining radishes on the side.

Nutritional analysis per serving: Calories: 340, Fat: 20 g, Saturated Fat: 4 g, Cholesterol: 130 mg, Fiber: 4 g, Protein: 27 g, Carbohydrates: 14 g, Sodium: 481 mg

TURKEY PICCATA WITH BRUSSELS SPROUT LEAVES AND BROCCOLI RABE

The capers are what make a piccata memorable—they're salty and pungent and stimulate your palate so that you enjoy all the fresh flavors of this dish. The traditional piccata is made from breadcrumb-coated veal escalopes, which takes away from the otherwise healthy nature of the dish. You can enjoy this updated version without sabotaging your health.

Serves: 4
Prep Time: 25 minutes
Cook Time: 25 minutes

- 2 bunches broccoli rabe (rapini) or kale, trimmed and cut into 5-cm pieces
- 450 g Brussels sprouts
- 4 tablespoons extra-virgin olive oil
- 3 garlic cloves, finely chopped
- sea salt and freshly ground black pepper
- 550 g thin-cut turkey breast steaks
- 2 tablespoons fresh lemon juice
- 1 tablespoon rinsed, finely chopped capers
- 2 tablespoons chopped fresh parsley

Bring a large saucepan of water to the boil over high heat. Cook the broccoli rabe until tender, about 3 minutes. Drain in a colander.

Remove the leaves of the Brussels sprouts by trimming the end of each one and halving it. Remove as many leaves as you can, saving the cores for vegetable stock. Reserve the leaves.

In a large nonstick sauté pan, warm 1 tablespoon of the oil over medium-high heat until shimmering. Cook the Brussels sprout leaves, stirring constantly, for about 6 minutes. Stir in the broccoli rabe and cook until the Brussels sprout leaves are tender, 2 to 3 minutes. Stir in the garlic, ¼ teaspoon salt, and a pinch of black pepper and cook for about 1 minute. Transfer the vegetables from the pan to a bowl; tent with foil to keep warm.

Wipe out the pan. Warm ½ tablespoon of the oil over medium–high heat until shimmering. Season the turkey with ¼ teaspoon each salt and black pepper. Sauté the turkey until browned and fully cooked, 2 to 3 minutes per side. Transfer the turkey to a platter.

Heat the remaining 2½ tablespoons oil over medium heat. Add the lemon juice, capers, and 1 tablespoon of water, stirring and using a spatula to scrape up any browned turkey bits in the pan. Spoon the mixture over the turkey breasts. Garnish with parsley and serve with the reserved vegetables on the side.

Nutritional analysis per serving: *Calories: 360, Fat: 16 g, Saturated Fat: 2.5 g, Cholesterol: 80 mg, Fiber: 6 g, Protein: 39 g, Carbohydrates: 17 g, Sodium: 470 mg*

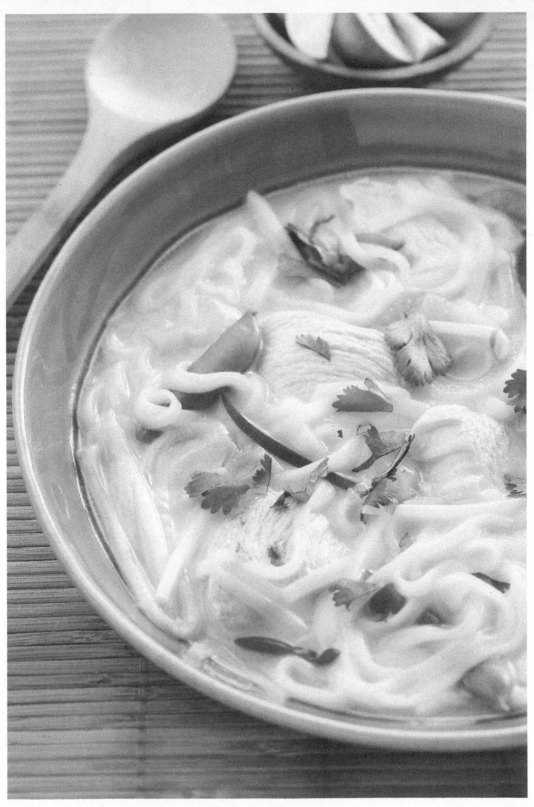

Thai Chicken Noodle Soup (page 130)

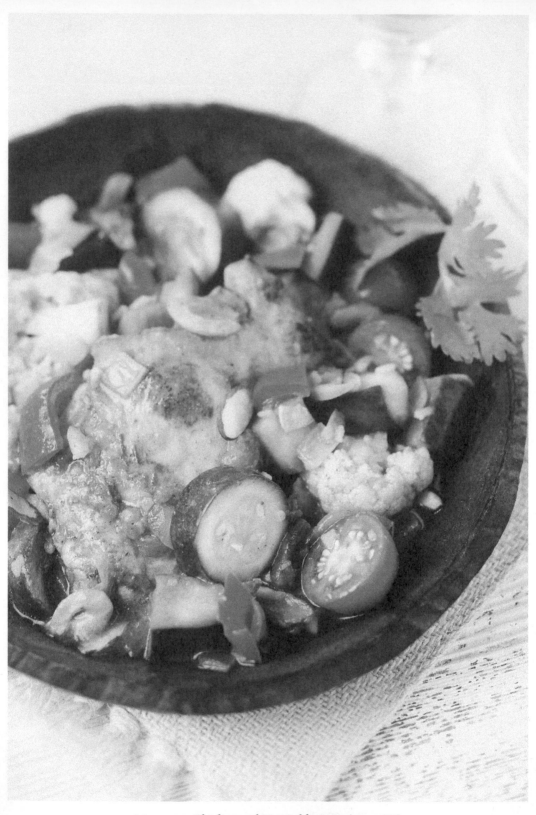

Moroccan Chicken and Vegetable Stew (page 175)

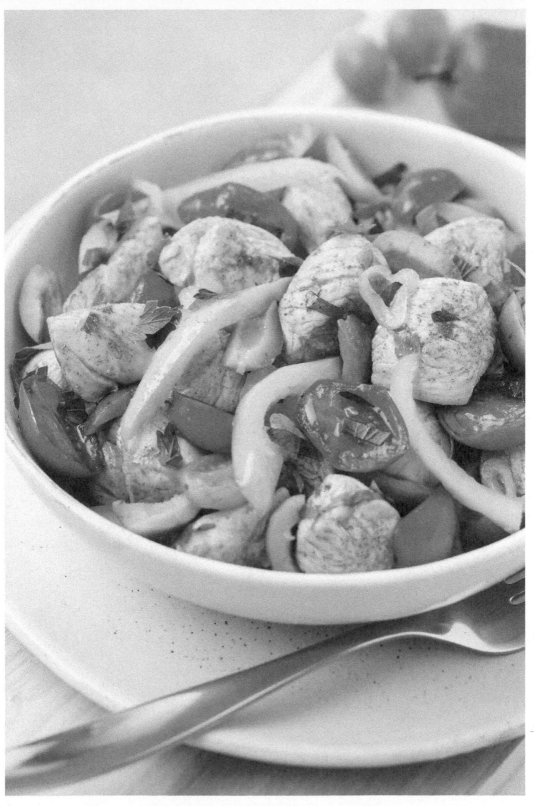

Chicken with Oven-Roasted Tomatoes (page 183)

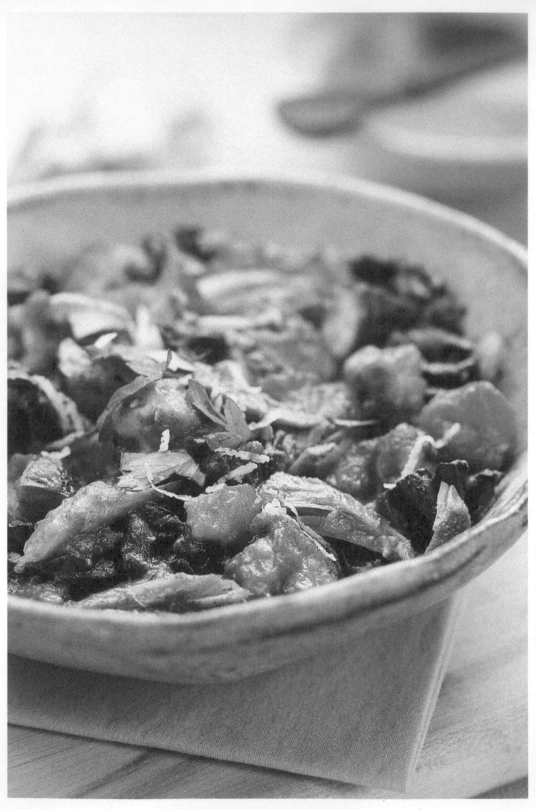

Lebanese-Style Lamb Stew (page 247)

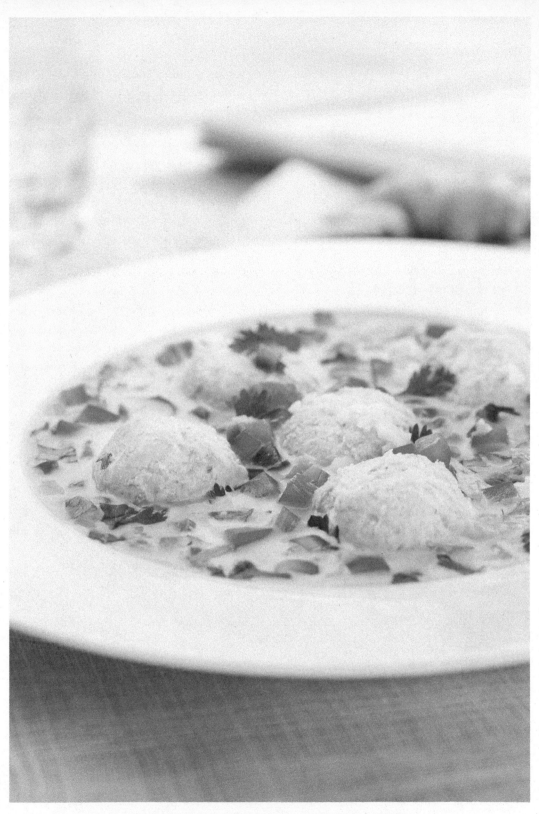

Yellow Curry with Chicken Meatballs (page 198)

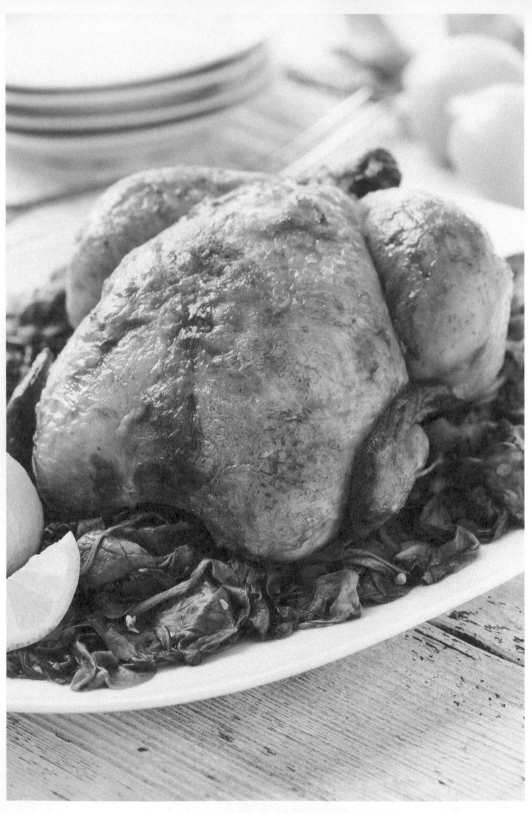

Ginger-Lemon Chicken with Spinach (page 202)

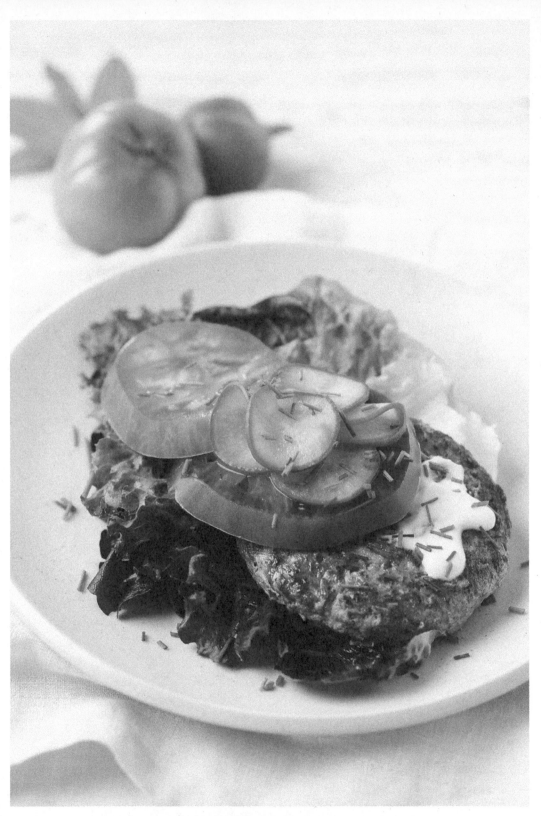

Turkey Burgers (page 213)

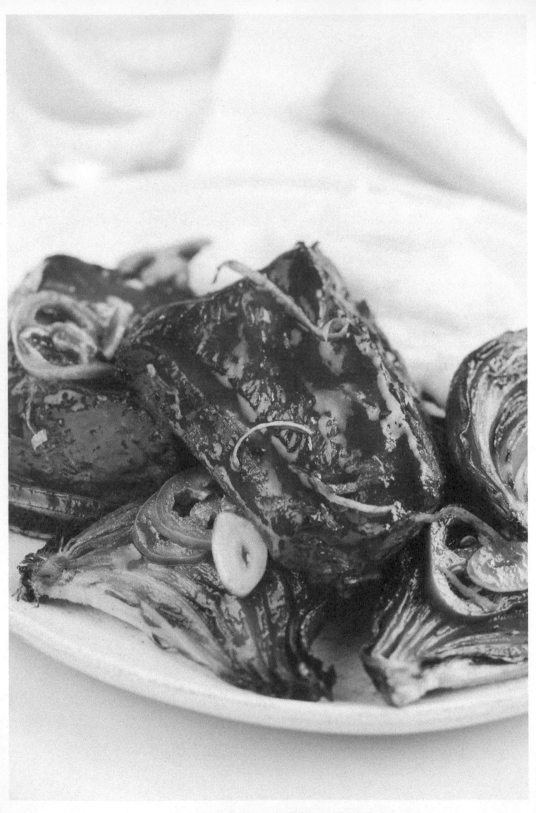

Slow-Cooked Short Ribs with Celeriac Puree (page 231)

Meat

BEEF CHILI

Higher in omega-3 fatty acids than grain-fed beef, as well as in other compounds known to reduce weight such as CLA (conjugated linoleic acids), 100% grass-fed beef is tasty and becoming more widely available as consumers increase demand for better quality meat.

Serves: 4
Prep Time: 30 minutes
Cook Time: 3 to 3½ hours

- 1 tablespoon extra-virgin olive oil
- 450 g grass-fed stewing steak, cut into 2.5-cm pieces
- 2 medium onions, chopped
- 2 green or red peppers, seeded and chopped
- 4 celery stalks, chopped
- 2 courgettes, diced
- 2 garlic cloves, finely chopped
- 1 tablespoon tomato puree
- 2 canned chipotle peppers in adobo sauce, seeded and chopped, plus 2 teaspoons adobo sauce
- 1 teaspoon ground cumin
- 1 teaspoon chili powder
- ½ teaspoon ground cinnamon
- ¼ teaspoon sea salt
- ¼ teaspoon freshly ground black pepper
- 2 (400-g) cans whole tomatoes
- 60 ml low-sodium chicken stock
- 20 g chopped fresh coriander, for garnish
- 30 g radishes, sliced, for garnish
- ½ avocado, stoned, peeled, and chopped, for garnish

In a cast-iron casserole, warm ½ tablespoon of the oil over medium-high heat until shimmering. Add the beef and cook until browned, about 3 minutes per side. Using a slotted spoon, transfer the beef to a bowl.

Add the remaining ½ tablespoon oil to the casserole. Sauté the onions and peppers for 6 minutes. Add the celery and courgettes and sauté for another 5 minutes. If the vegetables are browning too much, reduce the heat to medium.

Stir in the garlic, tomato puree, chipotle peppers, adobo sauce, cumin, chili powder, cinnamon, salt, and black pepper. Cook for 30 seconds before adding the tomatoes with their juices and the chicken stock. Use the back of a wooden spoon to break the tomatoes in half. Bring to the boil, then reduce the heat to low so the mixture is at a simmer.

Return the meat to the casserole, cover, and cook, stirring occasionally, until the meat is tender, 2½ to 3 hours. Taste and adjust the seasonings to make it spicier, if desired. Ladle the chili into bowls. Garnish with coriander, radishes, and avocado and serve.

Nutritional analysis per serving: Calories: 320, Fat: 11 g, Saturated Fat: 2.5 g, Cholesterol: 60 mg, Fiber: 8 g, Protein: 31 g, Carbohydrates: 26 g, Sodium: 310 mg

Slow-Cooked Brisket with Fennel and Onions

Make this a zero-fuss meal by prepping it Sunday night. Before leaving for the day on Monday morning, simply turn on your slow cooker and let the aroma of herbs, spices, and savory meat permeate your home. Walk in, enjoy the comforts of a truly slow-cooked meal, and marvel at the simplicity of living well. (If you don't have a slow cooker, you can cook the stew for about 1 hour in a covered cast-iron casserole set over medium heat.)

Serves: 4
Prep Time: 30 minutes
Cook Time: 8 to 10 hours (unattended), plus 10 minutes

- 2 tablespoons cider vinegar
- 2 fennel bulbs, halved and sliced
- 2 onions, halved and sliced
- 1 (400-g) can chopped tomatoes
- 1 head garlic, cloves peeled
- 8 to 10 thyme sprigs
- 1 (1.3-kg) grass-fed lean beef brisket joint, cut into 4 pieces
- 2 teaspoons chili powder
- ½ teaspoon sea salt
- ¼ teaspoon freshly ground black pepper
- chopped fresh parsley, for garnish

Pour the vinegar and 120 ml water into a 6-liter slow cooker.

In a large bowl, combine the fennel, onions, tomatoes with their juices, garlic, and thyme. Transfer half of the vegetable mixture to the slow cooker.

Season the brisket all over with the chili powder, salt, and black pepper. Place the pieces of meat on top of the vegetables in the slow cooker. Pour the remaining vegetables on top.

Cook on low until the meat easily pulls apart with a fork, 8 to 10 hours. Let the brisket rest, covered, for about 30 minutes. Remove the thyme sprigs.

Using a ladle, transfer 750 ml of the cooking liquid to a medium sauté pan. Bring to the boil over high heat and let the liquid reduce until it thickens into a gravy—keeping a careful eye on it so it doesn't over-reduce or burn—8 to 10 minutes. Remove from the heat.

Slice the brisket against the grain. Pour the gravy over the brisket slices, garnish with the parsley, and serve with the vegetables on the side.

Nutritional analysis per serving: *Calories: 300, Fat: 11 g, Saturated Fat: 4 g, Cholesterol: 76 mg, Fiber: 7 g, Protein: 27 g, Carbohydrates: 25 g, Sodium: 486 mg*

Asian-Style Beef Stew

Surprise your family with this Asian-style take on the traditional beef stew. It's comfort food at its tastiest — and healthiest.

Serves: 4
Prep Time: 15 minutes
Cook Time: 1 hour and 45 minutes

- 550 g grass-fed stewing steak, cut into 2.5-cm pieces
- 1 large daikon radish (mooli), peeled and cut into 2.5-cm pieces
- 4 spring onions, white parts cut into 5-cm lengths, green parts thinly sliced
- 2 tablespoons finely chopped fresh root ginger
- 3 tablespoons brown (*hatcho*) miso
- 2 small green courgettes, diced
- 2 small yellow courgettes, diced
- 200 g enoki mushrooms, trimmed and separated into smaller pieces
- ½ teaspoon freshly ground black pepper

Combine the beef, daikon, spring onion whites, and ginger in a large saucepan. Add 1 liter water; the water should just cover the ingredients. Bring to the boil over high heat. Skim and discard any foam that accumulates on the surface.

Meanwhile, whisk the miso with 120 ml warm water in a small bowl. Stir into the pan, reduce the heat to low, cover, and simmer until the beef is very tender, about 1½ hours.

Gently fold in the courgettes, mushrooms, and black pepper. Simmer until the courgettes are crisp-tender, about 10 minutes. Ladle into four soup bowls, garnish with the spring onion greens, and serve.

Nutritional analysis per serving: *Calories: 513, Fat: 28 g, Saturated Fat: 11 g, Cholesterol: 164 mg, Fiber: 5 g, Protein: 46 g, Carbohydrates: 19 g, Sodium: 551 mg*

Baked Meatballs with Cauliflower Puree

This is a sumptuous meal without the expense of a fancy restaurant! Feel free to substitute minced turkey for the beef in this recipe for a little variety.

Serves: 4
Prep Time: 30 minutes
Cook Time: 50 minutes

- 450 g minced grass-fed beef
- 4 button mushrooms, finely chopped
- 1 large omega-3 egg, beaten
- 6 garlic cloves, very finely chopped
- 1 shallot, finely chopped
- 2 tablespoons coarsely chopped pine nuts
- ½ teaspoon dried thyme
- ½ teaspoon dried oregano
- ½ teaspoon crushed chili flakes
- sea salt and freshly ground black pepper
- 2 tablespoons grapeseed oil
- 1 small cauliflower, coarsely chopped
- 4 tablespoons unsweetened almond milk
- 5 tablespoons extra-virgin olive oil
- 1 small onion, finely chopped
- 1 teaspoon tomato puree
- 500 ml passata
- 1 bunch kale, stems removed and finely shredded

Preheat the oven to 200°C/Gas 6.

In a large mixing bowl, combine the beef, mushrooms, egg, 2 teaspoons of the garlic, the shallot, pine nuts, thyme, oregano, chili flakes, ¼ teaspoon salt, and a pinch of black pepper. Mix well. Using wet hands, form the mixture into 12 balls, each about the size of a tangerine.

Heat the grapeseed oil in a large oven-proof sauté pan over medium-high heat until shimmering. Place the meatballs in the hot pan, leaving space between them. (Depending on the size of your sauté pan, you may need to cook the meatballs in batches.) Cook, using a large spoon to turn the meatballs gently, until brown, about 30 seconds per side. The meatballs will be soft, so turn carefully.

Transfer the sauté pan to the oven and bake until the meatballs feel firm to the touch, 8 to 10 minutes. Transfer them to a plate.

While the meatballs bake, pour 250 ml water into the bottom of a medium saucepan and bring it to the boil over high heat. Place a steaming rack or basket over the boiling water. Add the cauliflower, cover, and steam until it is very soft and easily breaks apart, about 10 minutes.

Transfer the cauliflower to a food processor or blender and add the almond milk, 4 tablespoons of the olive oil, and ¼ teaspoon salt. Puree until very smooth, then transfer the puree to a large oven-proof baking dish or gratin dish. Set aside.

In a large saucepan, heat the remaining 1 tablespoon olive oil over medium-low heat. Add the onion and remaining garlic and sauté until they begin to brown, about 5 minutes. Add the tomato puree and cook for 1 minute. Add the passata and ¼ teaspoon salt and bring to a simmer; reduce the heat to low and cook for 15 minutes. Stir in the shredded kale and cook until the kale is very tender, about 5 minutes.

Arrange the meatballs on top of the cauliflower puree, then ladle the tomato sauce over the meatballs. Place the baking dish in the oven and bake for 10 minutes.

Serve each guest 3 meatballs, along with some cauliflower puree and tomato-kale sauce.

Nutritional analysis per serving: *Calories: 499, Fat: 36 g, Saturated Fat: 6 g, Cholesterol: 140 mg, Fiber: 6 g, Protein: 29 g, Carbohydrates: 23 g, Sodium: 580 mg*

CHIPOTLE-RUBBED STEAK SALAD WITH ONIONS AND PEPPERS

Chipotle chilies are dried, smoked red jalapeños. If you can't find chipotle in powdered form, you can use ancho chili powder or smoked paprika.

Serves: 4
Prep Time: 20 minutes
Cook Time: 30 minutes

- 675 g grass-fed beef steaks (such as rib-eye or sirloin)
- 1 tablespoon chipotle chili powder
- 1 teaspoon sea salt
- ¼ teaspoon ground cumin
- ¼ teaspoon ground coriander
- 2 tablespoons extra-virgin olive oil
- 2 garlic cloves, finely chopped
- 3 small onions, sliced
- 3 peppers (mixed colors), seeded and thinly sliced
- 200 g baby rocket or mixed salad leaves

Pat the steaks dry with kitchen paper. In a small bowl, combine the chipotle powder, ½ teaspoon of the salt, the cumin, and the coriander. Rub the spice mixture all over the steaks and set aside.

In a large cast-iron frying pan or heavy sauté pan, heat 1 tablespoon of the olive oil over medium heat until shimmering. Add the garlic and onions and cook, stirring occasionally, until the onions are very soft and light golden brown, 10 to 12 minutes. Add the peppers and remaining ½ teaspoon salt and continue to cook until the peppers are very soft, another 8 to 10 minutes.

Line a large serving platter with the rocket. Remove the onions and peppers from the pan and arrange them over the rocket on the platter.

Rinse out the pan, then return it to the stove. Heat the remaining 1 tablespoon olive oil over high heat until shimmering. Place the steaks in the pan.

Cook the steaks for 4 minutes on one side, then flip and cook for another 4 minutes for medium-rare (internal temperature should be 135°F). Remove the steaks from the pan and allow them to rest for 10 minutes on a small rack set over a plate or baking tray to collect any juices.

Once the steaks have rested, transfer them to a chopping board and slice thinly against the grain. Arrange the sliced steak on top of the peppers on the platter, drizzle any accumulated juices over the meat, and serve.

Nutritional analysis per serving: *Calories: 360, Fat: 16 g, Saturated Fat: 3 g, Cholesterol: 94 mg, Fiber: 4 g, Protein: 42 g, Carbohydrates: 14 g, Sodium: 497 mg*

FILLET STEAK WITH GARLIC SAUCE AND ROASTED TOMATOES

The roasted tomatoes in this dish are excellent served warm, cold, or at room temperature—which is helpful when you have guests coming for dinner and you don't want to cook while entertaining.

Serves: 4
Prep Time: 15 minutes
Cook Time: 1 hour and 15 minutes

- 4 large heads garlic, unpeeled
- 4½ tablespoons extra-virgin olive oil
- 900 g cherry or baby plum tomatoes
- ¾ teaspoon sea salt
- ½ teaspoon freshly ground black pepper
- 2 tablespoons coconut oil
- 4 (2.5 to 3-cm-thick) fillet steaks
- 5 to 6 tablespoons low-sodium chicken stock
- 200 to 300 g baby rocket

Preheat the oven to 200°C/Gas 6.

Cut the top centimeter or so off each garlic head, just enough to expose the majority of the garlic cloves. Place each head on a large piece of foil. Drizzle ½ tablespoon of the olive oil over each head; wrap the foil around each head to enclose it in its own pouch.

Place the tomatoes on a large rimmed baking sheet. Drizzle with the remaining 2½ tablespoons olive oil and ¼ teaspoon each of the salt and black pepper and toss. Add the garlic pouches on the side of the baking sheet. Place the tomatoes and garlic in the preheated oven.

Roast the tomatoes until they burst and are caramelized, 45 to 60 minutes, making sure to stir midway through. Remove the garlic after about 50 minutes and let it sit until cool enough to handle. Tent the tomatoes with foil to keep warm.

Season the steaks with ¼ teaspoon each of the salt and black pepper. In a large cast-iron pan or oven-proof frying pan, heat the coconut oil over high heat until shimmering. Sear the steaks until golden brown on each side, about 5 minutes total. Transfer to the oven and cook until the steaks reach the desired internal temperature, about 8 minutes for medium-rare and 10 minutes for medium (a meat thermometer should register 54°C for medium-rare, 60°C for medium, and 71°C for well-done). Remove the steaks from the oven, tent with foil, and let rest for at least 5 minutes.

Meanwhile, grip the bottom of each garlic head and squeeze the roasted garlic into the bowl of a food processor. Add the remaining ¼ teaspoon salt and 5 tablespoons chicken stock. Puree until combined, adding another tablespoon of chicken stock if it is too thick. Transfer to a small saucepan and warm over low heat.

Place a steak on each plate, along with some of the roasted tomatoes. Drizzle the warm roasted garlic sauce over the steaks and serve.

Nutritional analysis per serving: *Calories: 490, Fat: 29 g, Saturated Fat: 8 g, Cholesterol: 120 mg, Fiber: 3 g, Protein: 43 g, Carbohydrates: 17 g, Sodium: 473 mg*

Rib-Eye Steaks with Grilled Radicchio

If you want to infuse a little sweetness into this savory meal, a touch of balsamic vinegar will do the trick.

Serves: 4
Prep Time: 10 minutes
Cook Time: 35 minutes

- 2 large heads radicchio, quartered lengthwise
- 4 tablespoons extra-virgin olive oil
- ½ teaspoon sea salt
- 675 g grass-fed boneless rib-eye steaks (5 cm thick)
- 450 g cherry tomatoes, halved
- 3 shallots, thinly sliced
- 4 tablespoons balsamic vinegar
- grated zest and juice of 1 lemon
- 2 garlic cloves, finely chopped

Preheat the oven to 250°C/Gas highest setting. In a large bowl, toss the radicchio with 2 tablespoons of the oil and ¼ teaspoon of the salt.

Heat a well-seasoned oven-proof griddle pan or large oven-proof frying pan over high heat. Cook 2 radicchio sections at a time, cut-side down, until the outer leaves are dark brown and crisp, 3 to 5 minutes per side. Transfer the radicchio to a chopping board and thinly slice crosswise.

Season the steaks with the remaining ¼ teaspoon salt. Place them in the pan and cook for 3 to 5 minutes per side. Transfer the pan to the oven and continue to cook the steaks for 6 to 8 minutes for medium (internal temperature should reach 60°C). Rest for 10 minutes before slicing.

Add the tomatoes, shallots, vinegar, lemon zest, and garlic to the hot pan. Allow the shallots and tomatoes to wilt slightly, 4 to 5 minutes. Remove from the heat and add the lemon juice. Add the radicchio to the pan and toss. Slice the steaks against the grain and serve over the salad.

Nutritional analysis per serving: *Calories: 540, Fat: 36 g, Saturated Fat: 13 g, Cholesterol: 116 mg, Fiber: 4 g, Protein: 36 g, Carbohydrates: 20 g, Sodium: 446 mg*

Herb-Crusted Beef Fillet

Take care not to overcook these steaks, as grass-fed beef tends to be leaner and will yield a tough and chewy steak when overdone.

Serves: 4
Prep Time: 30 minutes
Cook Time: 40 minutes

- 6 garlic cloves, 3 whole and 3 quartered
- 1 tablespoon plus 2 teaspoons extra-virgin olive oil
- 900 g baby plum or cherry tomatoes
- 1 fennel bulb, diced
- ½ teaspoon sea salt
- ½ teaspoon dried oregano
- ½ teaspoon dried thyme
- ½ teaspoon dried sage
- ¼ teaspoon finely chopped dried rosemary
- ¼ teaspoon freshly ground black pepper
- 1 tablespoon grapeseed oil
- 4 (175-g) grass-fed beef fillet steaks
- 1 large bunch asparagus, trimmed

Preheat the oven to 200°C. Place a rimmed baking sheet in the oven to preheat.

Place the 3 whole garlic cloves on a small piece of foil. Drizzle with 1 teaspoon of the olive oil and seal the garlic in the foil. Place the packet on the baking sheet. Remove the garlic after 15 minutes and confirm it is fully roasted—it will smell slightly sweet and feel soft. Set aside to cool. After the garlic has cooled, peel it and reserve.

While the garlic roasts, in a medium bowl, toss the tomatoes, fennel, the 3 quartered garlic cloves, 1 tablespoon of the olive oil, and ¼ teaspoon of the salt. Carefully distribute the vegetables over the preheated baking sheet and roast until the tomatoes are shriveling and beginning to brown, 35 to 40 minutes. When done, remove the vegetables from the baking sheet, place them in a bowl, and lightly crush the tomatoes with a fork.

In a small bowl, combine the whole roasted garlic cloves, oregano, thyme, sage, rosemary, black pepper, and remaining 1 teaspoon olive oil and mash with a fork to make a paste. Set aside.

Heat the grapeseed oil in a heavy cast-iron frying pan or oven-proof sauté pan over high heat until shimmering. Place the steaks in the pan, cook for 2 minutes, then flip and cook for another 2 minutes. While the second side cooks, spread 1 teaspoon of the garlic-herb paste over each steak. Transfer the pan to the oven and cook for 5 to 6 minutes for medium-rare (internal temperature 54°C), or 7 to 8 minutes for medium to medium-well (internal temperature 65°C). Allow the steaks to rest for 10 minutes.

While the steak rests, steam the asparagus: Pour 250 ml water into the bottom of a medium saucepan and bring it to the boil over high heat. Place a steaming rack or basket over the boiling water. Add the asparagus, cover, and steam until bright green and crisp-tender, 1 to 2 minutes. Divide the asparagus among four dinner plates. Top each plate with a steak and garnish with the roasted tomatoes and fennel.

Nutritional analysis per serving: Calories: 381, Fat: 20 g, Saturated Fat: 7 g, Cholesterol: 85 mg, Fiber: 5 g, Protein: 40 g, Carbohydrates: 15 g, Sodium: 418 mg

Slow-Cooked Short Ribs with Celeriac Puree

This is a great weekend meal; there's nothing difficult about it, nothing takes more than a half-hour of attention, and with the slow cooker going, you can come and go while dinner fixes itself. If you'd rather not use a slow cooker, bring the short ribs and other ingredients to the boil in a 5-liter cast-iron casserole over high heat. Transfer to a 180°C/Gas 4 oven and cook until the meat is falling off the bone, about 3 hours.

Serves: 6
Prep Time: 30 minutes
Cook Time: 4 hours (unattended), plus 1 hour

- 900 g bone-in beef short ribs, cut into 5-cm cubes by your butcher
- 120 ml balsamic vinegar
- 7 garlic cloves, 6 thinly sliced and 1 crushed
- 2 jalapeño chilies, seeded and sliced
- 2 tablespoons Dijon mustard
- grated zest of 2 lemons
- 2 teaspoons sea salt
- 3 large red onions, halved
- 1 celeriac, peeled and diced
- 1 (400-ml) can unsweetened coconut milk

Preheat the grill.

Line a rimmed baking sheet with foil and arrange the short ribs, meat-side up, evenly on the sheet. Place the baking sheet about 10 cm under the grill. Cook, turning the ribs occasionally, until each side is deep brown, 15 to 20 minutes total.

Combine 500 ml water, the vinegar, sliced garlic, jalapeños, mustard, lemon zest, and 1½ teaspoons of the salt in a 6-liter slow cooker. Add the ribs in an even layer. Cook on high for 4 hours. The meat should be tender when pierced with a fork.

Preheat the oven to 230°C/Gas 8.

With a slotted spoon, transfer the meat from the slow cooker to a plate.

Pour the cooking liquid into a gravy strainer to skim off the fat. Do not discard the fat (you should have about 4 tablespoons).

Add the skimmed cooking liquid to a medium saucepan. Cook over high heat until glossy and thickened and reduced to about 250 ml, 18 to 20 minutes. Remove from the heat. Moisten the short ribs with about 4 tablespoons of the sauce and set aside the rest to serve with the meal.

Meanwhile, on a large rimmed baking sheet, toss the onions with the reserved fat and the remaining ½ teaspoon salt. Arrange the onions, cut-side down. Roast, without turning, until the onions are browned on the underside, about 15 minutes. Flip and roast until the onions are tender, about 5 minutes more. Tent with foil and set aside.

Combine the celeriac, coconut milk, 250 ml water, and the crushed garlic in a 3-liter saucepan over medium heat. Bring to the boil, reduce the heat to low, and simmer, stirring occasionally, until the celeriac is very tender, 25 to 30 minutes.

Strain the celeriac, reserving the cooking liquid. Transfer the celeriac and about half of the cooking liquid to a blender. Blend with enough liquid to make a smooth puree, but not a sauce, scraping down the sides of the blender bowl frequently. If you have used all of the cooking liquid and your puree is still too thick, add a little water and continue to blend until it reaches the desired consistency. Transfer to a small saucepan and keep warm.

Serve the short ribs with the celeriac puree and roasted onions on the side, along with the gravy.

Nutritional analysis per serving: *Calories: 409 Fat: 31 g, Saturated Fat: 15 g, Cholesterol: 57 mg, Fiber: 3 g, Protein: 15 g, Carbohydrates: 18 g, Sodium: 467 mg*

SPICE-RUBBED BEEF FILLET WITH BRAISED GREEN BEANS AND MUSHROOMS

Enjoy these steaks with a side salad and Roasted Pepper and Red Onion Relish (page 298) for a sweet bite to accompany a savory meal. The leftover smoky-sweet spice rub for the beef can be used for other meats, fish, chicken, or vegetables.

Serves: 4
Prep Time: 15 minutes
Cook Time: 30 minutes

- 1 teaspoon ground turmeric
- 1 teaspoon sweet or smoked paprika
- 1 teaspoon ground coriander
- 1 teaspoon ground cumin
- 1 teaspoon ground ginger
- 1 teaspoon sea salt
- 4 (175-g) grass-fed fillet steaks
- 3 tablespoons extra-virgin olive oil
- 2 shallots, thinly sliced
- 225 g mixed mushrooms (such as button, chestnut, shiitake, and/or oyster), trimmed and thinly sliced
- 225 g green beans, trimmed and halved if large
- 250 ml low-sodium chicken stock
- 2 tablespoons apple cider vinegar

Preheat the oven to 200°C/Gas 6.

In a small bowl, combine the turmeric, paprika, coriander, cumin, ginger, and salt.

Pat the beef dry with kitchen paper, then sprinkle ¼ teaspoon of the spice rub on each steak and gently rub it all over the meat. Transfer the remaining spice rub to an airtight container and save for another use.

Heat 2 tablespoons of the olive oil in a large cast-iron frying pan or other heavy oven-proof sauté pan over high heat until shimmering. Place the steaks in the pan and cook for 1½ minutes, then flip the steaks and cook for another 1½ minutes. Transfer the pan to the oven and cook for 5 to 6 minutes for medium-rare (internal temperature 54°C), or 7 to 8 minutes for medium-well (internal temperature 65°C). Set aside the steaks to rest for 10 minutes before serving.

Wipe out the pan and place it over medium heat. Add the remaining 1 tablespoon olive oil and the shallots. Cook the shallots until they are fragrant and beginning to caramelize, about 3 minutes. Add the mushrooms and cook until they are softened and exuding their juices, 2 to 3 minutes. Add the green beans and cook for another minute.

Turn the heat to low, add the chicken stock and vinegar, and bring to a gentle simmer. Cook until the liquid has reduced by three-quarters and the beans are tender, 5 to 7 minutes.

To serve, distribute the braised beans and mushrooms among four plates and top each with a steak.

Nutritional analysis per serving: *Calories: 330, Fat: 17 g, Saturated Fat: 4 g, Cholesterol: 95 mg, Fiber: 2 g, Protein: 38 g, Carbohydrates: 12 g, Sodium: 532 mg*

BISON STEAKS WITH WILD MUSHROOM SAUCE AND FRENCH BEANS

Bison tend to be free-range, grass-fed, and wild for most of their life. This means that bison meat has a higher amount of anti-inflammatory omega-3 fatty acids and a better profile of saturated fats. Research shows that grass-fed meat is higher in stearic saturated fatty acids, which are heart-healthy and do not affect cholesterol levels.

Serves: 4
Prep Time: 20 minutes
Cook Time: 25 minutes

- 175 g fresh morels
- 115 g fresh shiitake mushrooms, stalks removed
- 2 large shallots, very thinly sliced
- 8 tablespoons grapeseed oil
- sea salt and freshly ground black pepper
- 450 g French beans, trimmed
- 4 (175-g) grass-fed bison rib-eye steaks
- 8 thyme sprigs, plus additional leaves for garnish
- 1 teaspoon fresh lemon juice
- 1 large omega-3 egg yolk

Preheat the oven to 200°C/Gas 6.

Swish the morels in a bowl of warm water to release all grit. Lift them out, and repeat two times. Cut the morels in half lengthwise. Cut the shiitake mushroom caps into pieces about the same size as the morels. Toss with half of the shallots, 2 tablespoons of the oil, and a pinch each of salt and black pepper on a large rimmed baking sheet. Spread in an even layer on one side of the baking sheet.

On the other side of the sheet, toss the French beans, remaining shallots, 1 tablespoon of the oil, ¼ teaspoon salt, and a pinch of black pepper. Spread in an even layer. Roast until the vegetables are tender, about 20 minutes. Remove from the oven and set aside.

Meanwhile, season the steaks with ½ teaspoon each salt and black pepper. Heat 2 tablespoons of the oil in a large oven-proof frying pan over medium-high heat until shimmering. Add the steaks to the pan and cook until well browned on the bottom, 1 to 2 minutes, then turn and cook until the other side is well browned, another 1 to 2 minutes. Scatter the thyme sprigs on top of the meat and transfer to the oven. Cook alongside the vegetables for 5 to 7 minutes for medium-rare (49°C). Discard the thyme sprigs. Transfer the steaks to serving plates and let them rest for 10 minutes.

Meanwhile, in a small saucepan, gently heat the remaining 3 tablespoons oil over low heat. Fill another saucepan with water and bring to a gentle simmer over medium-low heat. Set a medium bowl over the saucepan and in it whisk the lemon juice, egg yolk, 1 teaspoon of warm water, and ¼ teaspoon salt until thickened and warm. Continue whisking while adding the warmed oil from the other saucepan in a slow, steady stream. While still whisking, add 4 tablespoons of warm water in a slow, steady stream. Whisk until pale yellow, smooth, and creamy. Gently fold in the mushrooms from the baking sheet.

Spoon the mushrooms and sauce over and around the steaks. Place the French beans alongside the steaks. Garnish with thyme leaves and serve.

Nutritional analysis per serving: Calories: 480, Fat: 26 g, Saturated Fat: 4 g, Cholesterol: 150 mg, Fiber: 6 g, Protein: 43 g, Carbohydrates: 19 g, Sodium: 518 mg

Mexican "Rice" Bowl

Serve this fun, cheerful dish at your next family gathering to introduce the versatility and flavor that cooking with whole foods affords. This recipe incorporates cauliflower "rice" for a grain-free alternative.

Serves: 4
Prep Time: 20 minutes
Cook Time: 20 minutes

- 1 medium carrot, peeled
- 5 medium radishes
- ½ cucumber
- 2 spring onions, chopped
- 1½ to 2 tablespoons cider vinegar
- sea salt and freshly ground black pepper
- 2 tablespoons plus 1 teaspoon coconut oil
- 1 teaspoon finely chopped garlic
- 450 g minced grass-fed beef
- ½ teaspoon ground cumin
- ¼ teaspoon crushed chili flakes
- 1 cauliflower
- 1 small onion, finely chopped
- 1 avocado, stoned, peeled, and diced, for garnish
- 20 g chopped fresh coriander, for garnish
- lime wedges, for serving

Using a box grater, grate the carrot, radishes, and cucumber into a medium bowl. Mix in the spring onions, 1½ tablespoons of the vinegar, and ¼ teaspoon each salt and black pepper. Stir to combine; taste, adding ½ tablespoon more vinegar, if desired.

In a medium sauté pan, warm 1 teaspoon of the coconut oil over medium-high heat until shimmering. Add the garlic and cook, stirring constantly, for 30 seconds. Add the minced beef, along with the cumin, chili flakes, and ¼ teaspoon salt. Sauté, breaking up the beef with a wooden spoon, until fully cooked, 7 to 8 minutes. Transfer to a dish and tent with foil to keep warm.

Cut the cauliflower in half. Place a box grater over a large bowl and grate each cauliflower half over the big holes of the grater—hold the cauliflower by its stem as you grate it into "rice." Alternatively, you can coarsely chop the core and the florets and pulse them together in a food processor until they are reduced to the size of couscous or rice grains—be careful not to overprocess.

Heat the remaining 2 tablespoons coconut oil in a nonstick pan over medium-high heat until shimmering. Add the onion and cook until softened, 2 to 3 minutes. Add the cauliflower and combine. Cook, stirring frequently, until the cauliflower is slightly crispy on the outside but tender on the inside, 5 to 8 minutes. Season with a pinch of salt.

Divide the cauliflower "rice" among four bowls. Top each with beef and grated vegetables. Garnish with avocado and coriander and serve with lime wedges.

Nutritional analysis per serving: *Calories: 430, Fat: 30 g, Saturated Fat: 9 g, Cholesterol: 70 mg, Fiber: 8 g, Protein: 27 g, Carbohydrates: 17 g, Sodium: 430 mg*

Beef Bolognese

Try this take on Bolognese—but instead of serving over pasta, substitute low-carb shirataki noodles, which give this dish the traditional look and taste without all the extra carbs. Pair with Braised Broccoli with Tomatoes and Roasted Garlic (page 260).

Serves: 4
Prep Time: 20 minutes
Cook Time: 1 hour

- 1 tablespoon extra-virgin olive oil
- 450 g minced grass-fed beef
- 1 medium onion, finely chopped
- 300 g button mushrooms, trimmed and sliced
- 1 medium courgette, grated
- 2 garlic cloves, finely chopped
- 2 (400-g) cans choppd tomatoes
- ¾ teaspoon dried oregano
- ½ teaspoon dried thyme
- ½ teaspoon dried basil
- ½ teaspoon sea salt
- ¼ teaspoon freshly ground black pepper
- 2 bay leaves
- 2 (175 to 225-g) bags shirataki noodles, well rinsed
- 2 tablespoons chopped fresh basil, for garnish

In a medium saucepan, warm ½ tablespoon of the oil over medium–high heat until shimmering. Add the minced beef and sauté until it is fully cooked, about 8 minutes. Using a slotted spoon, transfer the meat to a bowl, leaving any oil in the pan.

Add the remaining ½ tablespoon oil to the pan. Add the onion and sauté until softened, about 8 minutes. Add the mushrooms and sauté until softened, 5 to 6 minutes. Stir in the grated courgette and sauté until wilted, another few minutes.

Add the garlic and cook, stirring, for 30 seconds. Add the chopped tomatoes with their juices, reserved minced beef, dried herbs, salt, black pepper, and bay leaves. Stir to combine. Let the sauce come to the boil and then reduce the heat to a simmer. Half cover with a lid and cook for 30 minutes. Remove the bay leaves.

Cook the shirataki noodles in boiling water according to the package directions. Transfer the cooked noodles to a colander. Blot the noodles dry with kitchen paper.

In a large bowl, toss the noodles with the meat sauce. Garnish with the fresh basil and serve.

Nutritional analysis per serving: Calories: 322, Fat: 17 g, Saturated Fat: 6 g, Cholesterol: 70 mg, Fiber: 5 g, Protein: 26 g, Carbohydrates: 18 g, Sodium: 397 mg

SUMMER PESTO "PASTA" WITH MINCED LAMB

Eating the 10-Day Detox way is not about restriction or deprivation — it's about healthful satisfaction. This meal replaces traditional flour-based pasta with courgette ribbons and features bright pesto flavors, giving you the feeling of a pasta-based meal without all the refined ingredients.

Serves: 4
Prep Time: 30 minutes
Cook Time: 15 minutes

- 50 g pine nuts
- 50 g fresh basil leaves
- 2 garlic cloves, halved
- 1 teaspoon sea salt
- ½ teaspoon freshly ground black pepper
- 2 tablespoons extra-virgin olive oil
- 5 large courgettes
- 450 g minced grass-fed lamb
- 2 medium tomatoes, chopped

In the bowl of a food processor, process the pine nuts until finely chopped, about 30 seconds. Add the basil leaves, garlic, and ¼ teaspoon each salt and black pepper and pulse until combined. Drizzle the olive oil and 1 tablespoon of water through the feed tube and continue to puree until a smooth consistency is achieved, scraping down the mixture as needed. Reserve the pesto.

Trim the ends of each courgette. Using a mandolin (or a vegetable peeler), slice the courgettes lengthwise into thin ribbons. Cut the ribbons in half crosswise so they don't tear while sautéing.

In a large nonstick sauté pan, sauté the lamb and ¼ teaspoon of the salt over medium-high heat until fully cooked, 6 to 8 minutes. Use a slotted spoon to transfer the meat to a bowl, leaving the juices from the lamb in the pan. Tent the meat with foil to keep warm.

Add half of the courgette ribbons to the drippings in the pan and sauté, stirring constantly, until the courgette is softened, 3 to 4 minutes. Transfer the courgettes to a large bowl. Repeat with the remaining courgette ribbons.

Use kitchen paper to blot excess moisture from the courgettes and season with the remaining ½ teaspoon salt and ¼ teaspoon black pepper. Top the courgettes with the pesto, lamb, and tomatoes. Using tongs, gently mix the ingredients to combine, and serve.

Nutritional analysis per serving: Calories: 570, Fat: 44 g, Saturated Fat: 15 g, Cholesterol: 85 mg, Fiber: 7 g, Protein: 26 g, Carbohydrates: 19 g, Sodium: 438 mg

LAMB AND CHARD STIR-FRY

Pair this dish with an appetizer like Creamy Herbed Tahini Dip with vegetables (page 281).

Serves: 4
Prep Time: 20 minutes
Cook Time: 10 minutes

- 1 tablespoon cumin seeds
- 1 teaspoon Szechuan or black peppercorns
- ½ teaspoon crushed chili flakes
- 2 tablespoons grapeseed oil
- 10 garlic cloves, thinly sliced
- 4 spring onions, thinly sliced, white and green parts separated
- 1 (550-g) boneless leg of grass-fed lamb, thinly sliced
- ¾ teaspoon sea salt
- 1 tablespoon gluten-free, low-sodium tamari
- 1 bunch Swiss chard or mustard greens, stems removed and chopped
- 1 tablespoon apple cider vinegar
- ½ jalapeño chili, seeded and very thinly sliced
- 4 tablespoons chopped fresh coriander

In a large frying pan, heat the cumin seeds and peppercorns over medium heat, tossing occasionally, until toasted, about 2 minutes. Cool, then transfer to a spice grinder, along with the chili flakes, and coarsely grind. Set aside.

Heat 1 tablespoon of the oil in the same pan over medium-high heat until shimmering. Add half of the garlic and half of the spring onion whites and cook, stirring, for 30 seconds. Add the lamb, sprinkle with half of the spice mix and ½ teaspoon of the salt, and cook, stirring occasionally, until browned, about 2 minutes. Stir in the tamari and transfer to a plate.

Add the remaining 1 tablespoon oil to the pan. Add the remaining garlic, spring onion whites, and spice mix. Cook, stirring, until just fragrant, about 1 minute. Add the chard and sprinkle with the remaining ¼ teaspoon salt. Cook, stirring, until the leaves are just wilted, about 2 minutes. Stir in the vinegar and the lamb with all its accumulated juices.

Transfer to a serving dish. Top with the spring onion greens, jalapeño, and coriander and serve.

Nutritional analysis per serving: *Calories: 290, Fat: 13 g, Saturated Fat: 3 g, Cholesterol: 90 mg, Fiber: 4 g, Protein: 33 g, Carbohydrates: 10 g, Sodium: 543 mg*

LAMB KORMA

Korma is a dish from northern India, typically made from lamb, cream, and sweet, toasty spices. Coconut milk is a great alternative for the dairy in this version. Adjust the cayenne to suit your heat preference; it's not typically a spicy dish, but feel free to crank up the heat if you like. Korma, like most stews, tastes better after a day or two in the refrigerator. Serve with a side of roasted cauliflower or Swiss chard.

Serves: 6
Prep Time: 15 minutes
Cook Time: 2 hours and 15 minutes

- 900 g grass-fed stewing lamb, cut into 2.5-cm pieces
- 1 teaspoon sea salt
- 2 tablespoons extra-virgin olive oil
- 1 medium onion, diced
- 8 garlic cloves, finely chopped
- 1 tablespoon grated fresh root ginger
- 2 teaspoons ground cumin
- 1 teaspoon ground coriander
- ½ teaspoon ground turmeric
- ½ teaspoon ground cinnamon
- ½ teaspoon cayenne pepper, or to taste
- ¼ teaspoon fennel seeds
- 225 g canned chopped tomatoes or diced fresh tomatoes with their juices
- 1 (400-ml) can full-fat unsweetened coconut milk
- 20 g chopped fresh coriander, for garnish

Preheat the oven to 180°C/Gas 4.

Pat the lamb dry with kitchen paper, then sprinkle with the salt. In a large oven-proof sauté pan or cast-iron casserole, heat the oil over high heat until shimmering. Working in batches if necessary so as not to crowd the pan, brown the lamb cubes all over, about 30 seconds per side.

Transfer the lamb to a plate and reduce the heat to medium. Add the onion, garlic, and ginger and cook until the onion begins to soften and become fragrant, 2 to 3 minutes, stirring constantly to avoid burning the garlic. Add the cumin, coriander, turmeric, cinnamon, cayenne, and fennel seeds and cook until the spices are fragrant, about 1 minute.

Return the lamb and any accumulated juices to the pan, and then add the tomatoes and coconut milk. Stir well, and bring to a simmer.

Cover the pan and transfer it to the oven. Cook for 1½ hours, then uncover the pan and continue to cook until the lamb is fork-tender, about 30 minutes more. If the sauce is getting very thick before the lamb is done, add 1 tablespoon of water at a time to reach the desired consistency.

Serve the lamb stew garnished with the coriander.

Nutritional analysis per serving: *Calories: 429, Fat: 26 g, Saturated Fat: 12 g, Cholesterol: 100 mg, Fiber: 1 g, Protein: 38 g, Carbohydrates: 8 g, Sodium: 491 mg*

LEBANESE-STYLE LAMB STEW

The texture and flavor of this hearty stew will keep your mouth happily entertained. Enjoy this robust dish the next time you crave comfort food.

Serves: 4
Prep Time: 20 minutes
Cook Time: 2 hours and 15 minutes

- 2 tablespoons extra-virgin olive oil
- 1.1 kg grass-fed lamb shanks
- sea salt and freshly ground black pepper
- 1 large onion, chopped
- 3 garlic cloves, thinly sliced
- 1 teaspoon ground ginger
- ½ teaspoon ground allspice
- ½ teaspoon ground cloves
- ½ teaspoon ground cinnamon
- ½ teaspoon freshly grated nutmeg
- 2 (400-g) cans whole tomatoes
- 900 g aubergines, trimmed and cut into 2-cm cubes
- 1 large bunch cavolo nero, tough stems removed, leaves sliced
- grated zest of 1 lemon
- 50 g fresh parsley, chopped
- lemon wedges, for serving

Heat 1 tablespoon of the oil in a large cast-iron casserole over medium-high heat until shimmering. Season the lamb with ½ teaspoon salt and ¼ teaspoon black pepper and add to the casserole. Cook, turning occasionally, until evenly browned, about 5 minutes. Transfer the lamb to a plate. Drain and discard the fat. Carefully wipe the pan clean with kitchen paper.

Heat the remaining 1 tablespoon oil in the same pan over medium heat. Add the onion and garlic, season with a pinch of salt, and stir well. Add 2 tablespoons of warm water and cook, stirring occasionally, until the onion is brown and crisp-tender, about 5 minutes. Add the ginger, allspice, cloves, cinnamon, and nutmeg. Cook, stirring, for 30 seconds. Add the tomatoes with their juices. Gently crush the tomatoes into small pieces with the back of a spoon. Return the lamb to the pan, nestle the meat in the mixture, and spoon the tomatoes on top. Cover, reduce the heat to low, and simmer for 1½ hours.

Meanwhile, dissolve 1½ teaspoons salt in 1.2 liters warm water in a large bowl. Add the aubergine pieces, weigh them down with a 15 to 20-cm plate, and soak for 30 minutes. Drain, rinse, and drain again.

After the lamb has simmered for 1½ hours, transfer the shanks to a plate, leaving the sauce in the pan. Stir the aubergine and cavolo nero into the pan. Simmer, uncovered, over low heat, stirring occasionally, until the aubergine is almost tender, about 20 minutes. When the lamb is cool enough to handle, pull the meat from the bones and discard the bones. Stir the meat into the pan and simmer until the aubergine is tender but still holding its shape, about 10 minutes. Stir in the lemon zest.

Season with ½ teaspoon each salt and black pepper and divide among four serving dishes. Sprinkle the parsley on top and serve with the lemon wedges.

Nutritional analysis per serving: Calories 440, Fat 17 g, Saturated Fat 4 g, Cholesterol 125 g, Fiber 13 g, Protein 41 g, Carbohydrate 35 g, Sodium 430 mg.

ROAST PORK FILLET WITH
COCONUT CURRY VEGETABLES

Shop at your local farmers' market during the summer months to procure vegetables at their peak for this dish. Fresh food has more flavor and nutrition—a win–win for your detoxification process. If you like a lot of heat, leave the seeds in the serrano chilies.

Serves: 4
Prep Time: 35 minutes
Cook Time: 1 hour

- 1 small aubergine, cut into 1-cm cubes
- 4 tablespoons plus 2 teaspoons extra-virgin olive oil
- sea salt
- 1 green courgette, halved lengthwise and cut into 1-cm-thick slices
- 1 yellow courgette, halved lengthwise and cut into 1-cm-thick slices
- 3 small onions, roughly chopped
- 2 or 3 serrano chilies, seeded and coarsely chopped
- 4 garlic cloves, halved
- 5-cm piece fresh root ginger, peeled and sliced
- 2 teaspoons garam masala
- 1 teaspoon ground turmeric
- 4 tablespoons coriander seeds
- 3 bay leaves
- 1 cinnamon stick
- 3 black cardamom pods
- 1 teaspoon cumin seeds
- 1 (400-g) can chopped tomatoes
- 160 ml unsweetened coconut cream
- juice of 2 lemons
- 20 g chopped fresh coriander, plus more for garnish
- 1 (675 g) pork fillet, halved lengthwise
- 2 tablespoons coconut oil
- ½ teaspoon ground cinnamon
- pinch of cayenne pepper

Preheat the oven to 250°C/Gas highest setting.

Line two rimmed baking sheets with foil. On one sheet, toss the auber-gine with 2 tablespoons of the olive oil and ¼ teaspoon salt. On the other sheet, toss the courgettes with 2 teaspoons of the olive oil and ¼ teaspoon salt. Roast, tossing occasionally and rotating the sheets halfway through, until the vegetables are tender and beginning to brown, 25 to 30 minutes. When the vegetables are done, preheat the grill.

Meanwhile, in the bowl of a food processor, process the onions, chil-ies, garlic, ginger, garam masala, turmeric, and 1¼ teaspoons salt into a thick paste. Set aside.

In an extra-large frying pan, combine the coriander seeds, bay leaves, cinnamon stick, cardamom pods, and cumin seeds. Over medium-high heat, cook the spices, stirring often, until fragrant, 2 to 3 minutes. Using a spice grinder (or clean coffee grinder), grind the mixture.

Add the remaining 2 tablespoons olive oil to the pan and heat over medium heat. Add the ground spice mixture and warm, stirring con-stantly, until the spices are fragrant, about 1 minute. Add the reserved onion paste and cook, stirring occasionally, until the paste is golden-brown, about 10 minutes.

Add the chopped tomatoes with their juices. Continue to cook, stir-ring occasionally, until the oil begins to separate and the paste becomes thinner and smoother, 10 to 12 minutes. Reserve 350 ml of the tomato mixture for the curry sauce and store any extra in a covered glass jar in the refrigerator for up to 3 days.

Add the coconut cream to the tomato mixture and raise the heat to medium-high until you reach a gentle simmer. Stir well.

Add the roasted aubergine and courgettes. Cook until the vegetables have absorbed some of the sauce and are completely tender, 6 to 8 min-utes. Stir in the lemon juice and coriander. Reduce the heat as low as pos-sible and cover to keep warm.

On a rimmed baking sheet lined with foil, brush the pork with the coconut oil, season with the ground cinnamon and cayenne, and sprinkle with a pinch of salt.

Grill the pork about 13 cm from the heat source, turning once, until the pork is fragrant and the spices are beginning to brown, 15 to 20 minutes; an instant-read thermometer inserted into the thickest part should register 65°C.

Slice the pork and divide it among four plates. Serve with some of the curry vegetable sauce.

Nutritional analysis per serving: *Calories: 547, Fat: 36 g, Saturated Fat: 18 g, Cholesterol: 87 mg, Fiber: 11 g, Protein: 315 g, Carbohydrates: 24 g, Sodium: 446 mg*

VEGETABLES AND SIDE DISHES

ROCKET AND FENNEL SALAD

Rocket is one of my favorite leaves. Here, the peppery zing of the rocket is matched perfectly with the slightly sweet crunch of the fennel. This salad will nicely complement any chicken, meat, or fish dish.

Serves: 4
Prep Time: 10 minutes

- 3 tablespoons extra-virgin olive oil
- juice of 1 lemon
- 2 small fennel bulbs, cored and thinly sliced
- 175 g baby rocket
- ¼ teaspoon sea salt
- pinch of freshly ground black pepper
- 2 tablespoons toasted pumpkin seeds, for garnish

In a large salad bowl, whisk the olive oil and lemon juice until combined. Add the sliced fennel and baby rocket. Season with the salt and black pepper and toss well. Garnish with toasted pumpkin seeds and serve.

Nutritional analysis per serving: *Calories: 170, Fat: 14 g, Saturated Fat: 2 g, Cholesterol: 0 mg, Fiber: 5 g, Protein: 4 g, Carbohydrates: 11 g, Sodium: 220 mg*

Heirloom Tomato, Cucumber, and Radish Salad

Heirloom tomatoes are old varieties that until recently were not widely grown or sold. Many of these beauties have been resurrected from obscurity and are unique in their colors, shapes, and widely varying flavors. If you can't find heirlooms, just use a mix of different tomatoes—whatever is freshest and ripest at your market. Never store tomatoes in the refrigerator; it destroys their flavor and stops them from further ripening.

Serves: 4
Prep Time: 10 minutes

- 450 g mixed heirloom tomatoes, cut into slices, wedges, and/or halves
- 1 small cucumber, thinly sliced
- 2 large radishes, thinly sliced
- 2 tablespoons flaked almonds
- 2 tablespoons extra-virgin olive oil
- ¼ teaspoon sea salt
- pinch of freshly ground black pepper
- 6 large fresh basil or mint leaves, thinly sliced

Arrange the tomatoes, cucumber, and radishes on a serving plate or on four individual plates. Sprinkle the almonds over the vegetables.

Drizzle the olive oil over the salad, then sprinkle with the salt, black pepper, and basil or mint. Serve.

Nutritional analysis per serving: *Calories: 100, Fat: 8 g, Saturated Fat: 1 g, Cholesterol: 0 mg, Fiber: 1 g, Protein: 2 g, Carbohydrates: 6 g, Sodium: 160 mg*

Green Beans and Almonds

Walnut and hazelnut oils are a true treat for your senses—not to mention your body. To maintain the phytonutrients and delicate healthy fats, select unrefined oil and store at room temperature for up to 6 months.

Serves: 4
Prep Time: 10 minutes
Cook Time: 5 minutes

- sea salt and freshly ground black pepper
- 675 g green beans, trimmed and halved
- 2 teaspoons Dijon mustard
- 2 teaspoons apple cider vinegar
- ½ shallot, finely chopped
- 1 garlic clove, finely chopped
- 2 tablespoons extra-virgin olive oil
- 1 tablespoon walnut or hazelnut oil
- 4 tablespoons flaked almonds

Bring a 5-liter saucepan of water to the boil over high heat. Add 1 tablespoon salt. Add the green beans and cook until crisp-tender, 3 to 4 minutes. Drain and immediately rinse with cold water.

Whisk together the mustard, vinegar, shallot, and garlic in a small bowl. Whisk in the olive and nut oils until combined. Season with a pinch each of salt and black pepper.

Drain the cooled beans and pat them dry, then transfer them to a serving bowl. Toss the beans with the dressing, and then gently mix in the almonds. Serve.

Nutritional analysis per serving: *Calories: 163, Fat: 10 g, Saturated Fat: 1 g, Cholesterol: 0 mg, Fiber: 6 g, Protein: 5 g, Carbohydrates: 17 g, Sodium: 185 mg*

SHREDDED BRUSSELS SPROUTS WITH WARM WALNUT DRESSING

Warming the dressing for this salad brings out the flavor of the mustard seeds and takes the raw edge off the shallot and garlic. It will also slightly wilt the shredded Brussels sprouts, allowing them to soak up the flavors and tenderize. Best of all, this salad can be served warm, at room temperature, or chilled.

Serves: 4
Prep Time: 15 minutes
Cook Time: 5 minutes

- 450 g Brussels sprouts, shredded
- 2 tablespoons grapeseed oil
- 2 tablespoons extra-virgin olive oil
- ½ shallot, finely chopped
- 1 garlic clove, finely chopped
- 1 teaspoon brown or black mustard seeds (if you can't find either, yellow is fine)
- 2 tablespoons apple cider vinegar
- ¼ teaspoon sea salt
- pinch of freshly ground black pepper
- 4 tablespoons chopped walnuts
- 1 tablespoon finely chopped fresh chives, for garnish (optional)

Pour 250 ml water into the bottom of a medium saucepan and bring it to the boil over high heat. Place a steaming rack or basket over the boiling water. Add the Brussels sprouts, cover, and steam until tender, 3 to 5 minutes. Transfer to a large bowl and allow them to cool.

In a small frying pan, heat both of the oils over low heat. Add the shallot, garlic, mustard seeds, vinegar, salt, and black pepper. When the dressing is slightly warm, drizzle it over the Brussels sprouts. Mix to coat evenly. Top with the walnuts and chives, if desired.

Nutritional analysis per serving: *Calories: 217, Fat: 19 g, Saturated Fat: 2 g, Cholesterol: 0 mg, Fiber: 4 g, Protein: 5 g, Carbohydrates: 11 g, Sodium: 168 mg*

Swiss Chard with Pine Nuts and Spring Onions

Chard and other leafy greens make great side dishes or bases for cooked vegetable salads. Chop up any leftover vegetables you have and serve them over sautéed greens, with a tasty vinaigrette. Add a poached or hard-boiled egg, some grilled fish, or a can of sardines for a complete meal.

Serves: 4
Prep Time: 15 minutes
Cook Time: 5 minutes

- 2 tablespoons extra-virgin olive oil
- 3 garlic cloves, finely chopped
- 1 large bunch Swiss chard, cut into 1-cm-wide strips
- 2 spring onions, thinly sliced
- 2 tablespoons pine nuts
- 2 teaspoons fresh lemon juice
- ½ teaspoon sea salt
- 4 tablespoons thinly sliced basil, for garnish (optional)

Heat a large sauté pan over medium heat until shimmering. Add the olive oil and garlic and cook for 1 minute.

Add the chard to the pan, increase the heat to high, and toss the chard to distribute the oil and garlic evenly. Cover the pan and cook for 1 minute.

Uncover the pan and continue to cook, stirring, until the chard is totally wilted and the juices in the pan fully evaporate, 3 to 4 minutes.

Scatter the spring onions and pine nuts over the chard, and sprinkle with lemon juice and salt. Serve garnished with basil, if desired.

Nutritional analysis per serving: *Calories: 113, Fat: 10 g, Saturated Fat: 1 g, Cholesterol: 0 mg, Fiber: 2 g, Protein: 3 g, Carbohydrates: 6 g, Sodium: 395 mg*

WILTED MIZUNA WITH WALNUTS

This recipe highlights the sweetness of coconut contrasted with the spicy greens.

Serves: 4
Prep Time: 5 minutes
Cook Time: 20 minutes

- sea salt
- 350 g green beans, trimmed
- 4 tablespoons unsweetened coconut flakes
- 3 tablespoons chopped walnuts
- 1 tablespoon coconut oil
- 1 tablespoon cumin seeds
- 1 tablespoon black or yellow mustard seeds
- 2 medium onions, finely chopped
- 1 tablespoon apple cider vinegar
- 350 g mizuna or rocket

Bring a large saucepan of water to the boil over high heat. Add 1 teaspoon salt. Add the green beans and cook just until they are crisp-tender, drain.

Meanwhile, toast the coconut flakes and walnuts in a large frying pan over medium heat, tossing occasionally, until golden brown and fragrant, about 5 minutes. Transfer to a plate and reserve.

Heat the oil in the same pan over medium heat. Add the cumin and mustard seeds and cook, stirring, until the seeds are fragrant and begin to pop, about 20 seconds. Add the onions and a pinch of salt and cook, stirring occasionally, until translucent and tender, about 7 minutes. Add the vinegar and cook until it has evaporated.

Add half of the mizuna and ¼ teaspoon salt. Cook, stirring, until wilted, about 2 minutes. Add the remaining mizuna, the green beans, and ¼ teaspoon salt. Fold gently until all of the mizuna is wilted. Transfer to a serving dish and top with the toasted walnuts and coconut flakes. Serve.

Nutritional analysis per serving: *Calories: 171, Fat: 12 g, Saturated Fat: 6 g, Cholesterol: 0 mg, Fiber 7 g, Protein: 6 g, Carbohydrates: 15 g, Sodium: 421 mg*

WILD MUSHROOM SAUTÉ

A simple yet delicious side with robust flavors—perfect over shirataki noodles or your favorite steamed vegetables.

Serves: 4
Prep Time: 15 minutes
Cook Time: 10 minutes

- 2 tablespoons extra-virgin olive oil
- 1 large shallot, finely chopped
- ¾ teaspoon sea salt
- 300 g maitake or shiitake mushrooms, trimmed and cut into 1-cm pieces
- 225 g oyster mushrooms, trimmed and cut into 1-cm pieces
- 150 g chestnut mushrooms, trimmed and cut into 1-cm pieces
- ¼ teaspoon freshly ground black pepper
- 1 teaspoon toasted sesame seeds
- grated zest and juice of 1 lime

Heat the oil in a large frying pan over medium-high heat until shimmering. Add the shallot and ¼ teaspoon of the salt. Cook until lightly browned, about 1 minute, stirring constantly.

Add the mushrooms, the remaining ½ teaspoon salt, and the black pepper. Cook until the mushrooms are brown and tender, about 8 minutes, stirring occasionally. The natural juices from the mushrooms will release and then evaporate.

Transfer the mushrooms to a serving platter and sprinkle with the sesame seeds, lime zest, and lime juice. Serve.

Nutritional analysis per serving: *Calories: 120, Fat: 8 g, Saturated Fat: 1 g, Cholesterol: 0 mg, Fiber: 4 g, Protein: 4 g, Carbohydrates: 12 g, Sodium: 418 mg*

Spicy Cauliflower Sauté

This side dish is so packed with flavor it will make a believer out of anyone who says vegetables are boring. Enjoy as a side dish or even as a snack or hors d'oeuvre at your next social gathering.

Serves: 4
Prep Time: 10 minutes
Cook Time: 40 minutes

- 4 tablespoons grapeseed oil
- 1 cauliflower, cored, florets cut into bite-size pieces
- 1 red pepper, seeded and sliced into 1-cm strips
- 2 jalapeño chilies, seeded and thinly sliced
- 3 garlic cloves, finely chopped
- 1 tablespoon gluten-free, low-sodium tamari
- lime wedges, for serving

In a large sauté pan, warm 2 tablespoons of the oil and 150 ml water over medium-high heat. Add half of the cauliflower and allow it to cook, stirring occasionally. After the water begins to evaporate and the cauliflower starts to fry in the oil, continue to stir until the cauliflower is brown and crisp, 6 to 8 minutes. Using a slotted spoon, transfer the cauliflower to a plate.

Cook the remaining cauliflower in the same way. During the last 2 minutes of cooking, add the red pepper, jalapeños, and garlic. Then return the first batch of cauliflower to the pan, add the tamari, and toss to combine.

Serve with lime wedges.

Nutritional analysis per serving: *Calories: 210 Fat: 15 g, Saturated Fat: 1.5 g, Cholesterol: 0 mg, Fiber: 7 g, Protein: 6 g, Carbohydrates: 18 g, Sodium: 260 mg*

Braised Broccoli with Tomatoes and Roasted Garlic

Serving whole broccoli spears makes for a creative way to enjoy broccoli.

Serves: 4
Prep Time: 10 minutes
Cook Time: 15 minutes

- 2 tablespoons extra-virgin olive oil
- 1 small red onion, thinly sliced
- 1 large head broccoli, cut into spears (see headnote)
- 2 tablespoons mashed Roasted Garlic with Olive Oil and Rosemary (page 287)
- 120 ml low-sodium chicken stock
- 300 g tomatoes, diced
- 1 tablespoon finely chopped fresh rosemary or ½ teaspoon dried rosemary
- ½ teaspoon sea salt
- pinch of freshly ground black pepper
- finely shredded fresh basil, for garnish (optional)

Heat the olive oil in a large sauté pan over medium heat until shimmering. Add the red onion and sauté until soft and beginning to brown, 3 to 5 minutes.

Add the broccoli and garlic paste and sauté for another minute, stirring to distribute the garlic throughout the broccoli.

Add the chicken stock, tomatoes, rosemary, salt, and black pepper and bring to a simmer. Reduce the heat to a low simmer, cover the pan, and cook for 5 minutes.

Uncover the pan, give the broccoli a good stir, and continue to cook, uncovered and stirring occasionally, until the liquid has mostly evaporated and the broccoli is quite soft, about 5 minutes. Garnish with basil, if desired, and serve.

Nutritional analysis per serving: *Calories: 120, Fat: 9 g, Saturated Fat: 1 g, Cholesterol: 5 mg, Fiber: 3 g, Protein: 3 g, Carbohydrates: 10 g, Sodium: 340 mg*

GARLIC AND CHILI TENDERSTEM BROCCOLI WITH SOFT-BOILED EGGS

Use any leftover broccoli in tomorrow's breakfast. Simply poach or boil an additional egg for more protein, sprinkle on a few chopped nuts for a little crunch, and serve with a side of berries.

Serves: 4
Prep Time: 25 minutes
Cook Time: 7 minutes

- 3 bunches tenderstem broccoli
- 4 garlic cloves, peeled
- 4 large omega-3 eggs
- 2 tablespoons extra-virgin olive oil
- ¾ tablespoon balsamic vinegar
- ¼ teaspoon crushed chili flakes
- ¼ teaspoon sea salt
- pinch of freshly ground black pepper

Bring a large saucepan of water to the boil over high heat.

While waiting for the water to boil, prepare the broccoli by trimming and discarding the bottom 2 cm of each stalk. Cut the stalks into 5-cm pieces, cutting thicker stalks in half lengthwise. Cut the tenderstem florets into bite-size pieces.

When the water is boiling, add the tenderstem stalks and garlic. Cook for 3 minutes. Add the florets, and cook for 1 minute. Transfer to a colander to drain, and run cold water over the broccoli and garlic to stop the cooking process.

To soft-boil the eggs, place them in a large saucepan and add enough cold water to cover by 2.5 cm. Bring to the boil over medium heat; then remove from the heat and cover. Let stand for 2 minutes. Transfer to a bowl with a slotted spoon and cover with cold water.

Remove the cooked garlic from the broccoli. Roughly chop the garlic and then mash it with a fork or the back of a knife. In a large bowl, combine the mashed garlic, olive oil, vinegar, chili flakes, salt, and black pepper.

Blot the broccoli with kitchen paper to remove any excess water. Add to the bowl with the dressing and toss to combine. Divide the broccoli among four plates. Carefully peel each egg and place on top of the broccoli. Serve.

Nutritional analysis per serving: Calories: 162, Fat: 12 g, Saturated Fat: 2 g, Cholesterol: 180 mg, Fiber: 3 g, Protein: 9 g, Carbohydrates: 7 g, Sodium: 234 mg

BROCCOLI RABE WITH HOT ITALIAN SAUSAGE

This dish is delicious served hot or cold, and may be enjoyed as a hearty snack, too. With a fried egg, it makes a great breakfast.

Serves: 4
Prep Time: 10 minutes
Cook Time: 10 minutes

- ¾ teaspoon sea salt
- 675 g broccoli rabe (rapini) or kale, trimmed of thick stems
- 2 tablespoons grapeseed oil
- 4 garlic cloves, thinly sliced
- 225 g hot Italian sausages
- grated zest and juice of 1 lemon
- lemon wedges, for serving

Bring a 3-liter saucepan of water to the boil over high heat. Prepare an ice bath by placing 6 ice cubes in a bowl and filling it to the top with cold water; set aside. Add ½ teaspoon salt and the broccoli rabe to the boiling water. Cook until just tender, 1 to 2 minutes. Drain, and transfer to the ice bath. When the broccoli has cooled, drain again and set aside.

Heat the oil in a large frying pan over high heat until shimmering. Add the garlic and cook, stirring constantly, until golden, about 20 seconds. Transfer the garlic to a plate and reserve. Add the sausage to the pan and sauté, breaking it up with the back of a spoon. Cook the sausage until it begins to brown and crisp, 3 to 4 minutes.

Add the broccoli rabe, lemon zest, and reserved garlic to the pan. Toss until warmed, 2 to 3 minutes, and season with the remaining ¼ teaspoon salt.

Transfer to a serving plate and sprinkle with the lemon juice. Serve immediately, with additional lemon wedges.

Nutritional analysis per serving: *Calories: 300, Fat: 25 g, Saturated Fat: 7 g, Cholesterol: 45 mg, Fiber: 4 g, Protein: 14 g, Carbohydrates: 7 g, Sodium: 495 mg*

Cauliflower "Rice"

This recipe is destined to become a family staple. You can adapt it to fit your taste preferences by changing up the seasonings and offering it with a variety of meals.

Serves: 4
Prep Time: 5 minutes
Cook Time: 10 minutes

- 1 cauliflower
- 2 tablespoons extra-virgin olive oil or coconut oil
- 1 small onion, finely chopped
- pinch of sea salt
- juice of ½ lime (optional)
- pinch of cumin (optional)
- 1 tablespoon chopped fresh coriander (optional)

Cut the cauliflower in half. Place a box grater over a large bowl and grate each cauliflower half over the big holes of the grater—hold the cauliflower by its stem as you grate it into "rice." Alternatively, you can coarsely chop the core and the florets and pulse them together in a food processor until they are reduced to the size of couscous or rice grains—be careful not to overprocess.

Heat the olive oil in a medium nonstick pan over medium-high heat until shimmering. Add the onion and cook until softened, 2 to 3 minutes.

Add the cauliflower "rice" to the pan and stir to combine. Cook, stirring frequently, until the cauliflower is slightly crispy on the outside but tender on the inside, 5 to 8 minutes. To enhance the flavor, add the lime juice, cumin, and/or coriander and serve.

Nutritional analysis per serving: *Calories: 84, Fat: 8 g, Saturated Fat: 1 g, Cholesterol: 0 mg, Fiber: 2 g, Protein: 1 g, Carbohydrates: 5 g, Sodium: 79 mg*

Mashed Cauliflower with Horseradish

It may be hard to believe that a rock-hard vegetable can be transformed into a soft, indulgent, and luscious treat, but this cauliflower preparation yields a texture reminiscent of the beloved mashed potato.

Serves: 4
Prep Time: 15 minutes
Cook Time: 20 minutes

- 2 tablespoons grapeseed oil
- ½ large Vidalia onion, finely chopped
- 1½ teaspoons sea salt
- 2 tablespoons pine nuts
- ½ teaspoon freshly grated nutmeg
- 1 cauliflower, stem trimmed and cut into 2.5-cm pieces
- 1 tablespoon freshly grated horseradish
- ¼ teaspoon freshly ground black pepper
- 1 tablespoon finely chopped fresh chives

Heat the oil in a small saucepan over medium-low heat. Add the onion and ¼ teaspoon of the salt and cook, stirring occasionally, until the onion is very tender but not browned, about 20 minutes. Stir in the pine nuts and nutmeg and cook for 1 more minute, stirring continuously to avoid burning the nuts.

Meanwhile, bring a large saucepan of water to the boil over high heat. Add 1 teaspoon of the salt. Cook the cauliflower until it is very tender, about 10 minutes. Drain and transfer to a food processor. Pulse until chopped.

Add the onion mixture to the food processor, along with the horseradish, black pepper, and remaining ¼ teaspoon salt. Pulse until almost completely smooth.

Transfer to a serving bowl, top with the chives, and serve.

Nutritional analysis per serving: *Calories: 200, Fat: 11 g, Saturated Fat: 1 g, Cholesterol: 0 mg, Fiber: 8 g, Protein: 7 g, Carbohydrates: 24 g, Sodium: 430 mg*

SPICY GARLIC AUBERGINE WITH MINT

I love the combination of spicy chili flakes and mint. Here, they balance each other beautifully with the neutral aubergine serving as the canvas to carry the flavors. Mint soothes the belly, so for those of you concerned about the spice in this dish, try it with a little extra mint.

Serves: 4
Prep Time: 15 minutes
Cook Time: 15 minutes

- 1½ tablespoons coconut oil
- 2 medium aubergines, diced
- ½ teaspoon sea salt
- ¼ teaspoon freshly ground black pepper
- 3 garlic cloves, finely chopped
- ½ teaspoon crushed chili flakes
- 10 fresh mint leaves, thinly sliced, for garnish

In a large nonstick sauté pan or frying pan, heat 1 tablespoon of the oil over medium-high heat until shimmering. Add as much of the aubergines as you can fit in the pan, probably about two-thirds, and cook for 3 to 4 minutes, stirring constantly. As the aubergines shrink a bit, stir in the remaining aubergine, along with the salt and black pepper. Continue sautéing and stirring until the aubergine is tender, 6 to 7 more minutes.

Next, push a bit of aubergine to the side of the pan. Add the remaining ½ tablespoon oil, along with the garlic and chili flakes. Stir until the garlic is cooked, 30 seconds to 1 minute. Then, stir to combine with the aubergine. Garnish the aubergine with mint and serve.

Nutritional analysis per serving: *Calories: 120, Fat: 6 g, Saturated Fat: 4.5 g, Cholesterol: 0 mg, Fiber: 8 g, Protein: 3 g, Carbohydrates: 17 g, Sodium: 300 mg*

STEAMED VEGETABLES WITH LEMON AIOLI

Making aioli is very rewarding, as you transform simple ingredients into a new, unrecognizable form. Dollop on poached eggs for a nice breakfast treat.

Serves: 8
Prep Time: 15 minutes
Cook Time: 10 minutes

- 1 large omega-3 egg yolk
- grated zest of ½ lemon
- 1 garlic clove, halved
- ¼ teaspoon sea salt
- 120 ml extra-virgin olive oil
- 450 g asparagus, trimmed
- 225 g mangetout, trimmed
- 1 large summer squash (courgette, spaghetti or pattypan squash) cut into 1-cm-thick spears
- 1 red pepper, seeded and cut into 5-mm-thick strips

Combine the egg yolk, lemon zest, garlic, salt, and 1 teaspoon of water in the bowl of a food processor. Pulse a few times; then, with the machine running, stream the oil in through the feed tube and blend until all of the oil is incorporated and the aioli is smooth. Transfer to a small bowl.

Pour 250 ml water into the bottom of a medium saucepan and bring it to the boil over high heat. Place a steaming rack or basket over the boiling water. Add the asparagus, cover, and steam until bright green and crisp-tender, about 4 minutes. Transfer the asparagus to a platter large enough for all of the vegetables, but keep the water boiling. Steam the mangetout until bright green and crisp-tender, about 2 minutes. Transfer to the platter. Steam the squash until crisp-tender, about 3 minutes.

Add the red pepper strips to the platter of steamed vegetables and serve with the aioli on the side, for dipping.

Nutritional analysis per serving: *Calories: 150, Fat: 15 g, Saturated Fat: 2 g, Cholesterol: 28 mg, Fiber: 3 g, Protein: 4 g, Carbohydrates: 17 g, Sodium: 87 mg*

Courgette Ribbons with Pearl Onions and Cardamom

Pearl, or baby, onions are sweet and mild. They're usually sold unpeeled, but some stores now carry them peeled, which makes this dish even faster and easier to prepare (you can just skip the blanching step). This side dish can be served hot, at room temperature, or chilled—making it a versatile addition to your bag of culinary tricks.

Serves: 4
Prep Time: 10 minutes
Cook Time: 15 minutes

- 10 pearl onions
- 2 tablespoons extra-virgin olive oil
- 1 small shallot, thinly sliced
- 1 teaspoon grated fresh root ginger
- 120 ml low-sodium chicken stock
- ½ teaspoon sea salt
- 1 courgette, shaved (with a mandolin or vegetable peeler) into long ribbons
- 2 tablespoons flaked almonds or chopped hazelnuts
- 1 tablespoon thinly sliced fresh mint leaves
- ¼ teaspoon ground cardamom

Bring a large saucepan of water to the boil over high heat. Prepare an ice bath by placing 6 ice cubes in a bowl and filling it to the top with cold water; set aside. Blanch the onions in the boiling water for 1 to 2 minutes. Remove them from the water and transfer them to the ice bath. Drain them after a couple of minutes, and then you should be able to easily remove the skins.

Heat the olive oil in a large sauté pan over medium heat until shimmering. Add the shallot and sauté gently until soft and beginning to brown, about 2 minutes. Add the ginger and pearl onions and sauté until the onions begin to brown slightly, about 5 minutes.

Add the chicken stock and salt and bring to a gentle simmer, cover the pan, and cook until the stock has completely evaporated, about 5 minutes. Remove the pan from the heat.

Add the courgette, almonds, mint, and cardamom and toss well to combine and to allow the courgette to wilt from the residual heat in the pan. Serve.

Nutritional analysis per serving: *Calories: 118, Fat: 9 g, Saturated Fat: 1 g, Cholesterol: 0 mg, Fiber: 2 g, Protein: 2 g, Carbohydrates: 10 g, Sodium: 306 mg*

Braised Celery Hearts in Walnut Oil

While it's great to have a variety of oils to cook with, for this recipe it is fine to substitute another nut oil or additional extra-virgin olive oil if you don't happen to have walnut oil on hand.

Serves: 4
Prep Time: 5 minutes
Cook Time: 25 minutes

- 450 g organic celery
- 2 tablespoons extra-virgin olive oil
- 1 garlic clove, finely chopped
- 1 bay leaf
- ¼ teaspoon sea salt
- pinch of freshly ground black pepper
- 1 tablespoon walnut oil

Use a vegetable peeler to peel the outer skin off the celery stalks. Trim both ends and cut the hearts in half crosswise.

Warm the olive oil in a large frying pan over medium heat until shimmering. Add the celery and cook, turning occasionally, until golden brown on all sides, 8 to 10 minutes. Add 250 ml water, the garlic, bay leaf, salt, and black pepper. Cover and cook until most of the liquid has evaporated and the celery is tender, 14 to 15 minutes.

Discard the bay leaf and serve the celery drizzled with the walnut oil.

Nutritional analysis per serving: *Calories: 110, Fat: 10 g, Saturated Fat: 1.5 g, Cholesterol: 0 mg, Fiber: 2 g, Protein: 0 g, Carbohydrates: 4 g, Sodium: 270 mg*

JICAMA FRIES

Jicama is a nonstarchy root vegetable commonly used in Mexico and Southeast Asia. It has a crisp, juicy texture and a slightly sweet flavor. Use it raw in salads and slaws, or cooked in place of starchier root vegetables.

Serves: 4
Prep Time: 10 minutes
Cook Time: 35 minutes

- 1 large jicama, peeled and cut into 5-mm sticks
- 1 tablespoon extra-virgin olive oil
- ¼ teaspoon sea salt
- pinch of freshly ground black pepper
- ¼ teaspoon smoked or sweet paprika (optional)
- ¼ teaspoon ground cumin (optional)

Preheat the oven to 200°C. Place a large rimmed baking sheet in the oven to preheat.

In a bowl, toss the jicama sticks with the olive oil, salt, black pepper, and spices, if desired.

Carefully spread the jicama sticks onto the hot baking sheet in a single layer. Roast for 20 minutes; then, give them a stir and roast for another 15 minutes. Serve hot.

Nutritional analysis per serving: *Calories: 145, Fat: 4 g, Saturated Fat: 1 g, Cholesterol: 0 mg, Fiber: 15 g, Protein: 2 g, Carbohydrates: 27 g, Sodium: 157 mg*

SNACKS

CUCUMBER-KALE SMOOTHIE

Enjoy this smoothie as a refreshing afternoon pick-me-up to keep you energized and focused. Having a small protein-based snack between 2 p.m. and 4 p.m. helps regulate blood sugar levels and the hormones that keep your body's circadian clock in a comfortable rhythm.

Serves: 1
Prep Time: 10 minutes

- 10-cm piece cucumber, peeled
- 20 g kale leaves
- 2 raw walnuts
- 2.5-cm piece fresh root ginger, peeled and coarsely chopped
- 2 tablespoons almond butter
- 175 ml unsweetened almond milk
- 1 tablespoon fresh lemon juice
- 1 tablespoon chia seeds
- 2 large ice cubes

Combine all of the ingredients in a blender and blend on high speed until smooth, 1 to 2 minutes. If the smoothie is too thick, add a little water and blend again until it reaches the desired consistency. Drink immediately.

Nutritional analysis per serving: *Calories: 376, Fat: 30 g, Saturated Fat: 4 g, Cholesterol: 0 mg, Fiber: 9 g, Protein: 14 g, Carbohydrates: 17 g, Sodium: 148 mg*

SPICY MOCKTAIL

This is the spicy afternoon counterpart to your morning vegetable smoothie, with a touch of tofu for added protein.

Serves: 1
Prep Time: 20 minutes

- 25 g spinach leaves
- ½ tomato, chopped
- 2 celery stalks
- 3 radishes, chopped
- 115 g non-GMO silken or soft tofu
- 1 teaspoon fresh lemon juice
- pinch of cayenne pepper, or to taste
- pinch of freshly ground black pepper
- pinch of celery salt
- 2 ice cubes

Place all of the ingredients, except for one celery stalk, in a blender and puree until blended, 30 seconds to 1 minute, stopping to scrape down the blender if necessary. Taste and adjust the seasonings as desired.

Pour into a glass. Garnish with the celery stalk and serve.

Nutritional analysis per serving: *Calories: 95, Fat: 4 g, Saturated Fat: 1 g, Cholesterol: 0 mg, Fiber: 4 g, Protein: 7 g, Carbohydrates: 9 g, Sodium: 248 mg*

DEVILED EGGS

Dress up your normal hard-boiled version with this creative twist on deviled eggs. The incredible egg is a power food because it contains phytonutrients, complete protein, and healthy fats. It makes for an ideal low-glycemic afternoon snack.

Serves: 4
Prep Time: 20 minutes
Cook Time: 5 minutes

- 1 small summer squash (courgette or pattypan), coarsely grated
- ½ teaspoon sea salt
- 4 large omega-3 eggs
- 1 spring onion, finely chopped
- 2 tablespoons tahini
- 1 tablespoon Mayonnaise (page 299) or Vegenaise
- 2 teaspoons fresh lemon juice
- sesame seeds, for garnish
- cayenne pepper, or smoked or sweet paprika, for garnish

Place the squash in a colander, sprinkle with ¼ teaspoon of the salt, and set the colander in the sink to drain the excess liquid.

Put the eggs in a large saucepan and add enough cold water to cover by 2.5 cm. Bring to the boil over medium-high heat, remove from the heat, and cover. Let stand for 12 minutes. Transfer the eggs to a bowl with a slotted spoon and cover with cold water. When cold, peel the eggs and cut each in half lengthwise. Scoop out the yolks and place them in a small bowl.

Squeeze as much liquid as possible out of the squash. Add the squash, spring onion (reserving some of the greens for garnish), tahini, mayonnaise, and lemon juice to the bowl with the egg yolks. Mix until well combined and season with the remaining ¼ teaspoon salt.

Divide the yolk mixture among the egg white halves. Sprinkle the tops with the reserved spring onion greens, sesame seeds, and cayenne pepper, and serve.

Nutritional analysis per serving: *Calories 133, Fat 10 g, Saturated Fat 2 g, Cholesterol 226 mg, Fiber 1 g, Protein 9 g, Carbohydrates 5 g, Sodium 383 mg*

EGG SALAD IN CHICORY SPEARS

chicory is a slightly bitter vegetable that looks like a small, elongated, pale yellow-green lettuce. The individual leaves are great for holding dips, spreads, and salads. If chicory isn't available, you can also use the smaller inner leaves of romaine lettuce, or scoop the egg salad onto cucumber rounds.

Serves: 4
Prep Time: 15 minutes
Cook Time: 5 minutes

- 2 large omega-3 eggs
- 1 celery stalk, including leaves, finely diced
- 1 spring onion, finely sliced
- 1 tablespoon finely chopped fresh chives, basil, or parsley
- 2 tablespoons Mayonnaise (page 299) or Vegenaise
- 2 teaspoons Dijon or grainy French mustard
- ½ teaspoon ground turmeric
- ¼ teaspoon smoked or sweet paprika
- sea salt and freshly ground black pepper
- 1 head chicory, leaves separated

Put the eggs in a large saucepan and add enough cold water to cover by 2.5 cm. Bring to the boil over medium-high heat, remove from the heat, and cover. Let stand for 12 minutes. Transfer to a bowl with a slotted spoon and cover with cold water. When cold, peel the eggs and dice.

In a small bowl, combine the diced eggs, celery, spring onion, and chives and mix gently with a fork. Add the mayonnaise, mustard, turmeric, and paprika and combine. Season with salt and black pepper to taste.

Scoop the egg salad onto the chicory leaves and serve.

Nutritional analysis per serving: *Calories: 90, Fat: 8 g, Saturated Fat: 1.5 g, Cholesterol: 95 mg, Fiber: 1 g, Protein: 3 g, Carbohydrates: 2 g, Sodium: 290 mg*

Stuffed Tomatoes

I love growing tomatoes in my summer garden. There is nothing better than inviting a group of friends over to enjoy a bike ride and an afternoon snack featuring homegrown vegetables. You don't have to have a garden to enjoy this recipe with your friends—you just have to appreciate delicious, easy, and satisfying snack foods.

Serves: 4
Prep Time: 20 minutes
Cook Time: 5 minutes

- 2 poblano peppers
- 8 medium tomatoes
- 1 avocado, peeled and stoned
- ½ bunch coriander, including stems
- 1½ teaspoons fresh lime juice
- ½ teaspoon sea salt
- 2 tablespoons toasted sunflower seeds

Rest the peppers on the hob of a gas stove. Turn the flame to medium and char the peppers, turning them with tongs, until evenly blackened and blistered, about 5 minutes. (Alternatively, you can roast the peppers under the grill.) Transfer to a bowl, cover with clingfilm, and let steam. When cool enough to handle, rub off the charred skin and discard, along with the stems and seeds.

While the peppers cool, slice off a little from the top and bottom of each tomato to create flat surfaces. Cut the tomatoes in half. Scoop out and discard the seeds.

Transfer the peppers to a food processor, along with the avocado, coriander, lime juice, and salt. Puree until very smooth. Transfer to a zip-lock plastic bag and snip a hole in one corner. Pipe the avocado mixture into the tomato halves. Top with the sunflower seeds and serve.

Nutritional analysis per serving: *Calories: 140, Fat: 9 g, Saturated Fat: 1.5 g, Cholesterol: 0 mg, Fiber: 4 g, Protein: 2 g, Carbohydrates: 12 g, Sodium: 300 mg*

PEPPER MINI QUICHES

I make a double batch of these quiches and freeze half. That way, on busy mornings when I am catching a plane or need a snack between meetings, I can pop one in my toaster oven and avoid craving something sweet.

Serves: 12
Prep Time: 10 minutes
Cook Time: 20 minutes

- 1 tablespoon grapeseed oil
- 8 large omega-3 eggs
- 4 peppers (yellow, green, and red), seeded and finely chopped
- 1 teaspoon sea salt
- ½ teaspoon cumin
- ¼ teaspoon freshly ground black pepper
- pinch of cayenne pepper, or to taste

Preheat the oven to 230°C/Gas 8. Brush a 12-cup muffin tin with the grapeseed oil.

Whisk the eggs in a large bowl. Add the peppers, salt, cumin, black pepper, and cayenne and stir to combine. Divide the egg mixture among the muffin cups, filling them just below the rim. Place the muffin tin on a rimmed baking sheet and transfer it to the oven.

Bake, rotating once, until the quiches are puffy and brown and a cocktail stick inserted into the center comes out clean, 18 to 20 minutes. Serve warm.

Store leftovers in an airtight container in the refrigerator for up to 3 days. Simply reheat in the oven at 170°C/Gas 3 until warmed through, about 10 minutes.

Nutritional analysis per serving (1 mini quiche): *Calories 145, Fat 9 g, Saturated Fat 2 g, Cholesterol 300 mg, Fiber 2 g, Protein 11 g, Carbohydrates 8 g, Sodium 586 mg*

ROASTED VEGETABLES WITH ARTICHOKE HUMMUS

Artichokes are one of my favorite vegetables because they peak during the winter, yet there is something very light and springlike about them. This twist on hummus substitutes artichokes for chickpeas to yield that creaminess we all love. Along with great flavor and texture, this recipe boasts healthy amounts of fiber and is sure to satisfy you for hours until your next meal.

Serves: 8
Prep Time: 15 minutes
Cook Time: 30 minutes

- 1 large cauliflower, cored and cut into 5-cm florets
- 150 ml extra-virgin olive oil
- 450 g asparagus, trimmed
- 225 g green beans, trimmed
- 300 g Brussels sprouts, trimmed and halved
- 300 g cherry tomatoes
- 500 g frozen artichoke hearts, thawed
- 2 garlic cloves, halved
- 4 tablespoons tahini
- grated zest and juice of 1 lemon
- 1 tablespoon chopped fresh parsley
- ½ teaspoon sea salt
- ¼ teaspoon freshly ground black pepper
- ¼ teaspoon ground cumin

Preheat the oven to 230°C. Line two rimmed baking sheets with foil.

In a large bowl, toss the cauliflower with 2 tablespoons of the oil. Transfer the cauliflower to one of the lined baking sheets and roast until tender, 15 to 20 minutes. Place half of the cauliflower in a food processor and the other half on a platter.

Toss the asparagus, green beans, Brussels sprouts, and tomatoes with 4 tablespoons of the olive oil and divide between the two lined baking sheets. Roast until the vegetables are crisp-tender and beginning to brown,

10 to 15 minutes. Transfer to the platter with the cauliflower and let cool.

Meanwhile, to the food processor add the artichoke hearts, garlic, tahini, lemon zest and juice, and the remaining olive oil. Puree, scraping down the sides occasionally, until smooth. Add the parsley, salt, black pepper, and cumin and continue to puree until well combined.

Serve the roasted vegetables with the artichoke dip. Store any leftover dip in an airtight container in the refrigerator for up to 5 days.

Nutritional analysis per serving: *Calories: 290, Fat: 22 g, Saturated Fat: 3.5 g, Cholesterol: 0 mg, Fiber: 10 g, Protein: 7 g, Carbohydrates: 20 g, Sodium: 160 mg*

SARDINE-CUCUMBER BITES

Sardines are a good source of omega–3 fatty acids without the mercury levels seen in larger fish. Enjoy a bit of the olive oil they are packed in for extra healthy fat.

Serves: 4
Prep Time: 20 minutes

- 2 tablespoons fresh lemon juice
- 1 tablespoon Mayonnaise (page 299) or Vegenaise
- 2 tablespoons finely chopped fresh chives, plus more for garnish
- 1 tablespoon capers, rinsed, drained, and chopped
- 1 teaspoon smoked paprika, plus more for garnish
- 1 (200-g) can oil-packed wild sardines, flaked into small pieces, oil reserved
- 1 small red pepper, seeded and finely chopped
- 1 cucumber, trimmed and sliced

Combine the lemon juice, mayonnaise, chives, capers, and paprika in a large bowl.

Fold in the sardines and red pepper and gently mix. Add 1 tablespoon of oil from the sardine can if the mixture is dry.

Mound the sardine mixture onto the cucumber slices and garnish with additional paprika. Serve.

Nutritional analysis per serving: *Calories: 140 Fat: 8 g, Saturated Fat: 1 g, Cholesterol: 70 mg, Fiber: 1 g, Protein: 13 g, Carbohydrates: 4 g, Sodium: 340 mg*

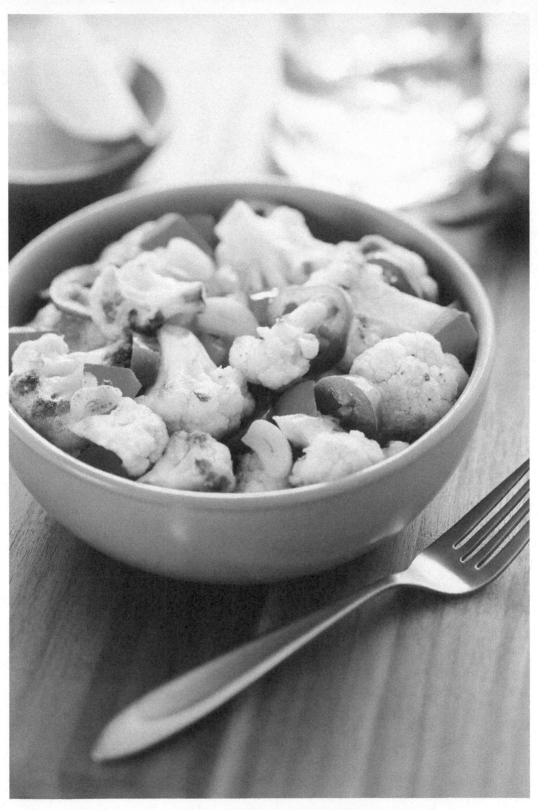

Spicy Cauliflower Sauté (page 259)

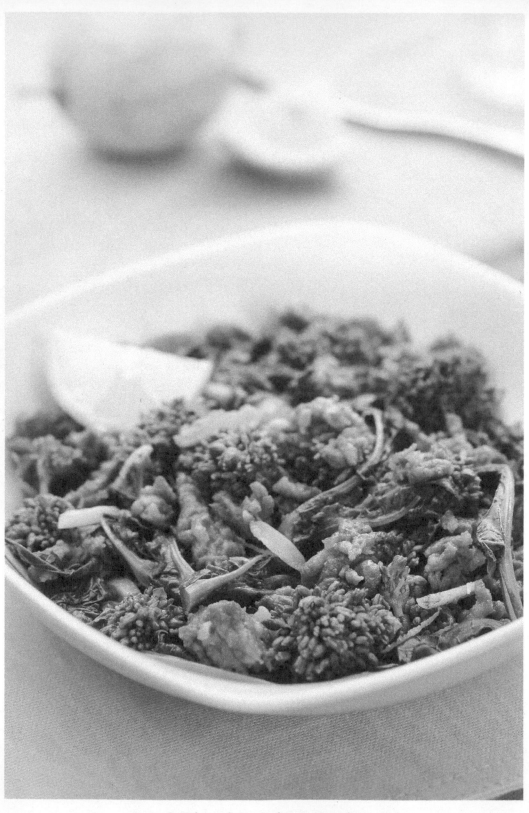

Broccoli Rabe with Hot Italian Sausage (page 263)

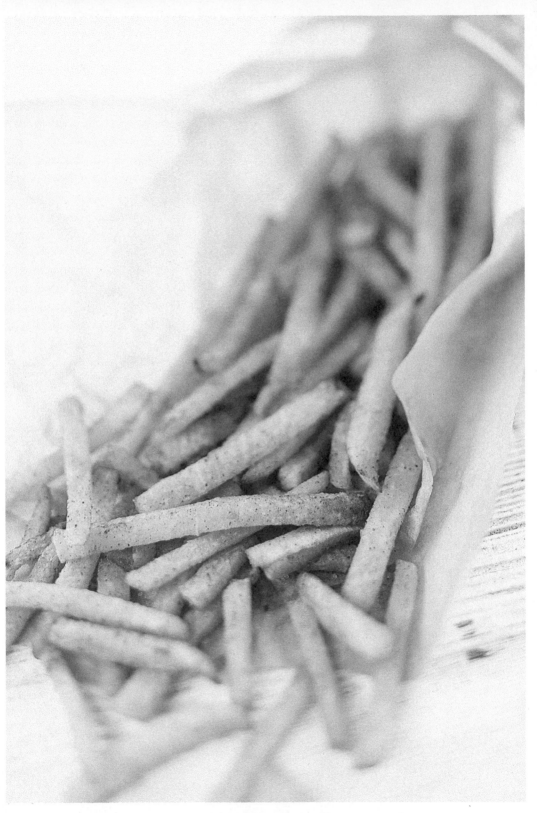
Jicama Fries (page 271)

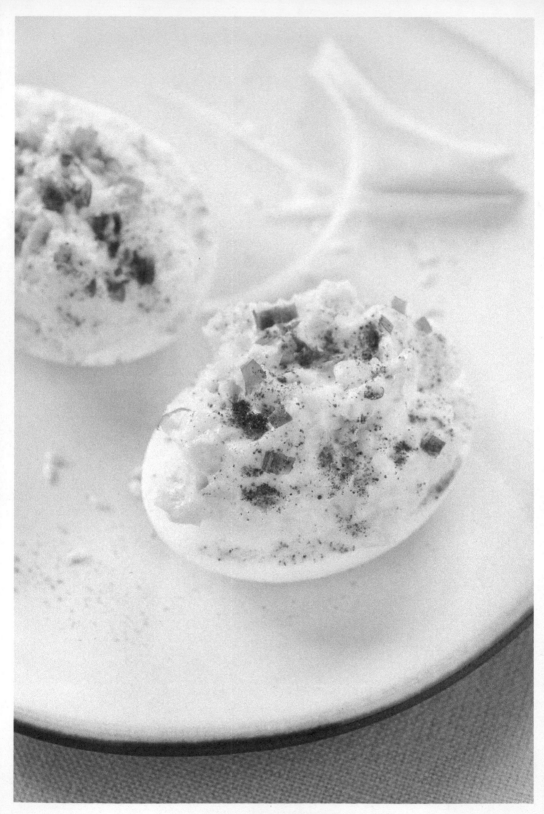

Deviled Eggs (page 274)

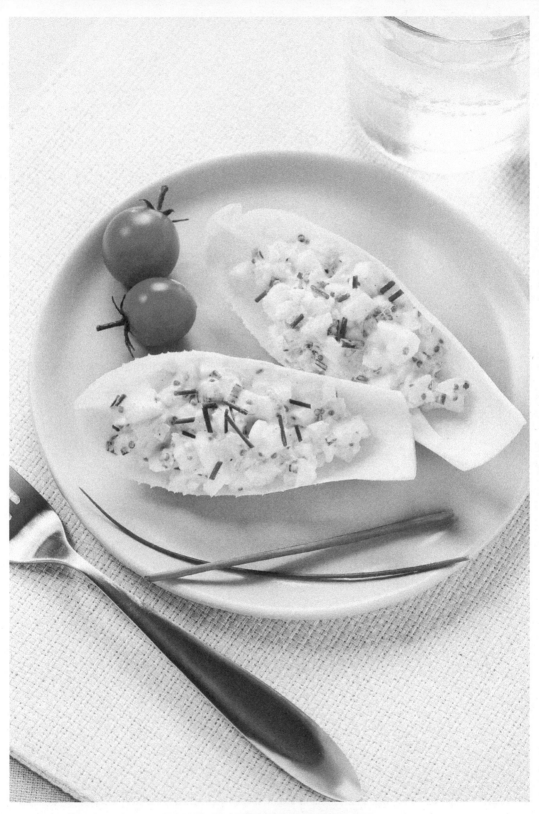

Egg Salad in Chicory Spears (page 275)

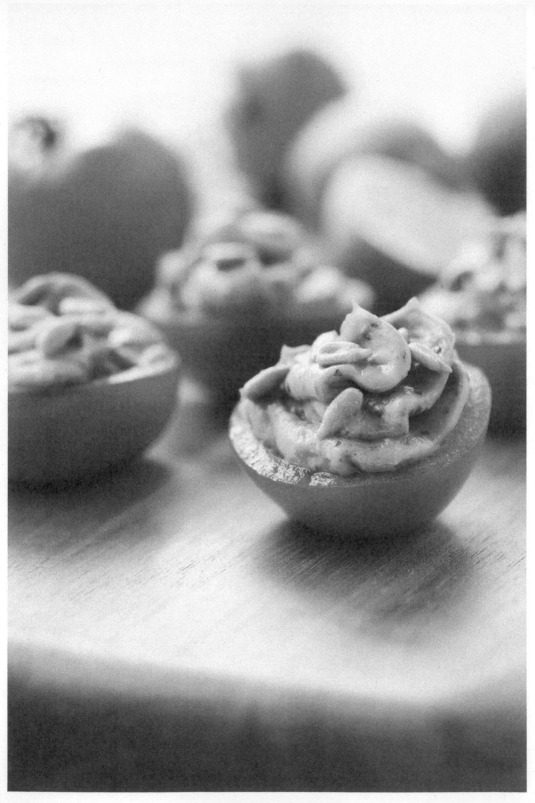

Stuffed Tomatoes (page 276)

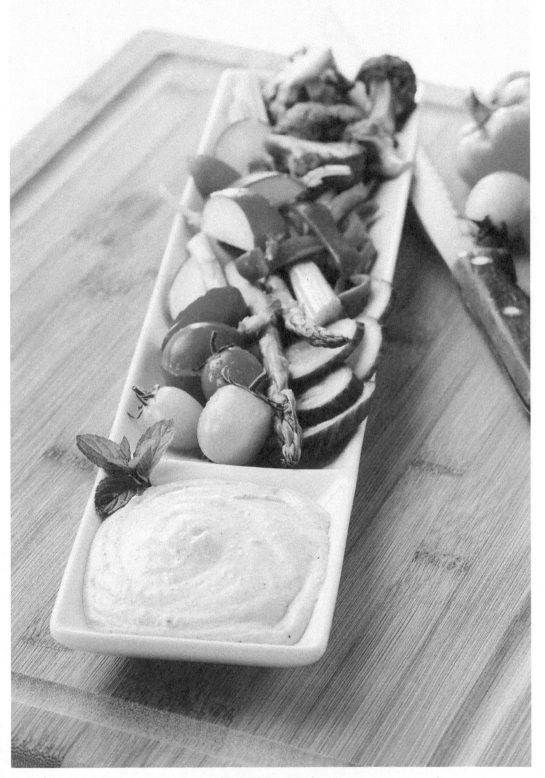

Creamy Herbed Tahini Dip (page 281)

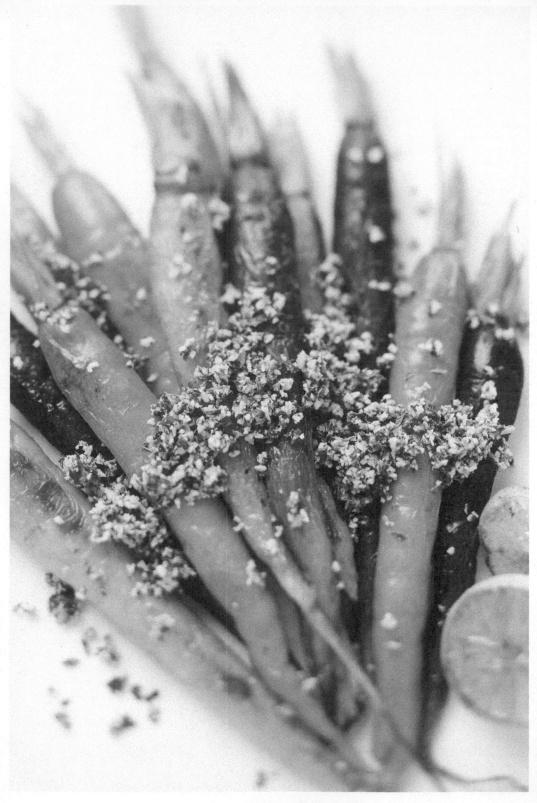

Gremolata with Almonds (page 292)

CREAMY HERBED TAHINI DIP

Tahini is a key ingredient in hummus and falafel, and is also used to make many other sauces and dips. It's rich, creamy, and very nutritious. Serve this dip with raw vegetables (such as celery, cucumber, cherry tomatoes, broccoli, mangetout, tenderstem broccoli, and French beans) or as a sauce over grilled fish.

Makes: about 500 ml
Prep Time: 15 minutes

- 250 ml tahini
- 4 tablespoons fresh coriander leaves
- 8 to 10 fresh mint leaves
- 5 large fresh basil leaves
- 1 large spring onion, cut into 5-cm pieces
- 2 tablespoons finely chopped fresh chives
- 1 garlic clove, halved
- juice of 1 lemon
- 2 tablespoons extra-virgin olive oil
- ½ teaspoon sea salt
- ¼ teaspoon ground turmeric
- ¼ teaspoon ground cumin
- ¼ teaspoon ground coriander
- ¼ teaspoon fennel or anise seeds

Combine all of the ingredients plus 250 ml hot water in a blender and blend until smooth. Add more hot water as needed if the blender is struggling. Serve.

Store any leftover dip in an airtight container in the refrigerator for up to 5 days.

Nutritional analysis per serving (2 tablespoons): *Calories: 105, Fat: 10 g, Saturated Fat: 1 g, Cholesterol: 0 mg, Fiber: 1 g, Protein: 3 g, Carbohydrates: 4 g, Sodium: 79 mg*

Spicy Roasted Pepper and Walnut Dip

Here's a great snack to serve with carrots, radishes, sugar snap peas, celery, jicama, or any other favorite crunchy fresh vegetable.

Makes: about 500 ml
Prep Time: 10 minutes
Cook Time: 30 minutes

- 2 tablespoons extra-virgin olive oil
- 4 red peppers, seeded and cut into 1-cm-thick strips
- 4 tablespoons shelled walnuts
- ½ to ¾ teaspoon crushed chili flakes
- ¼ teaspoon sea salt

Preheat the oven to 260°C/Gas highest setting.

Line two rimmed baking sheets with aluminium foil and brush with the oil. Spread the red peppers out on the sheets and roast until they are tender and browning at the edges, 17 to 20 minutes.

Transfer the peppers to a food processor and process until smooth. Add the walnuts, crushed chili flakes, and salt and process again until smooth. Serve.

Store any leftover dip in an airtight container in the refrigerator for up to 5 days.

Nutritional analysis per serving (4 tablespoons): *Calories: 70, Fat: 6 g, Saturated Fat: 0.5 g, Cholesterol: 0 mg, Fiber: 1 g, Protein: 1 g, Carbohydrates: 4 g, Sodium: 75 mg*

BABA GHANOUSH

Baba ghanoush is a traditional Middle Eastern aubergine dip.

Serves: 8
Prep Time: 10 minutes, plus cooling time
Cook Time: 55 minutes

- 2 small aubergines
- 4 tablespoons tahini
- 2 tablespoons extra-virgin olive oil
- 2 garlic cloves, halved
- juice of 1 lemon
- ½ teaspoon sea salt
- 4 tablespoons coarsely chopped parsley
- 1 bunch celery, cut into sticks, for serving

Preheat the grill. Line a rimmed baking sheet with foil.

Prick each aubergine a few times with a fork and place on the lined baking sheet. Place the aubergines about 10 cm under the grill and grill, turning every 5 minutes or so, until the skin is completely charred, 15 to 20 minutes. Remove from the grill and heat the oven to 190°C/Gas 5.

When the oven comes to temperature, return the aubergines to the oven and roast until they are completely soft, 30 to 35 minutes; when pressed with the back of a fork they should offer little resistance.

Allow the aubergines to cool enough so that you can handle them, about 25 minutes. Cut each aubergine in half and, using a rubber spatula, carefully scrape out the pulp. Discard the skin.

In a blender or food processor, combine the aubergine pulp, tahini, olive oil, garlic, lemon juice, and salt. Puree until smooth. Transfer the dip to a serving bowl and stir in the parsley. Serve with celery sticks for dipping.

Store any leftovers in an airtight container in the fridge for up to 5 days.

Nutritional analysis per serving (4 tablespoons): *Calories: 120, Fat: 8 g, Saturated Fat: 1 g, Cholesterol: 0 mg, Fiber: 5 g, Protein: 3 g, Carbohydrates: 12 g, Sodium: 240 mg*

WARM HERBED OLIVES

Try to find olives that have not been pitted, as they generally taste better and are of higher quality than pitted olives.

Serves: 8
Prep Time: 10 minutes

- 120 ml extra-virgin olive oil
- 2 garlic cloves, lightly crushed
- 5-cm strip lemon peel
- 1 bay leaf
- 6 to 8 black peppercorns
- ½ teaspoon dried rosemary or thyme
- ½ teaspoon fennel seeds
- 350 g mixed unpitted olives

In a small saucepan, combine all of the ingredients except the olives. Over very low heat, warm the oil just until the garlic starts to gently sizzle, then remove from the heat.

Place the olives in a glass or ceramic bowl and pour the warm oil over them. Allow the olives to marinate at room temperature for 1 hour before serving.

Store any leftover olives in an airtight container in the refrigerator for up to 2 weeks; allow to come to room temperature before serving.

Nutritional analysis per serving (4 tablespoons): *Calories: 159, Fat: 16 g, Saturated Fat: 2 g, Cholesterol: 0 mg, Fiber: 1 g, Protein: 1 g, Carbohydrates: 4 g, Sodium: 517 mg*

Gua-Kale-Mole

If you have picky eaters around, this recipe is one you will want to whip up soon! They won't even know they are eating healthy greens with each delicious, delectable bite. Serve with fresh veggie dippers such as cucumbers, radishes, sugar snap peas, cherry tomatoes, cauliflowers, red peppers, and carrots.

Serves: 6
Prep Time: 15 minutes

- 2 bunches kale, stems removed and roughly chopped
- 1 bunch coriander, stems included
- 1/33 tomatoes, chopped
- 1/3 red onion, chopped
- 1 jalapeño chili, seeded and halved
- 1 garlic clove, halved
- juice of 2 limes
- ½ teaspoon sea salt
- 3 avocados, peeled and stoned

In the bowl of a food processor, combine the kale, coriander, two-thirds of the chopped tomato, 1½ tablespoons of the onion, the jalapeño, garlic, lime juice, and salt. Puree the mixture until smooth, scraping down the sides as needed, 1 to 2 minutes. Add the avocados and puree again until blended, 30 seconds to 1 minute.

Transfer the gua-kale-mole to a bowl and stir in the remaining chopped tomatoes and onion. Serve.

Store any leftover dip in an airtight container, with greaseproof paper pressed against the surface to prevent discoloration, in the refrigerator for up to 5 days.

Nutritional analysis per serving (120 ml): *Calories: 216, Fat: 15 g, Saturated Fat: 2 g, Cholesterol: 0 mg, Fiber: 10 g, Protein: 6 g, Carbohydrates: 20 g, Sodium: 235 mg*

CINNAMON AND CAYENNE ROASTED MIXED NUTS

Try this sweet and spicy version of roasted nuts in place of your normal mid-morning snack.

Serves: 18
Prep Time: 10 minutes
Cook Time: 30 minutes

- 175 g raw pecan halves
- 200 g raw cashews
- 200 g raw almonds
- 3 tablespoons coconut oil
- 1½ teaspoons ground cinnamon
- 1 teaspoon ground sweet paprika
- ½ to 1 teaspoon cayenne pepper
- ½ teaspoon sea salt
- ¼ teaspoon freshly ground black pepper

Preheat the oven to 180°C/Gas 4. Line a baking sheet with aluminium foil.

In a large bowl, combine the pecans, cashews, and almonds. In a small bowl, combine the coconut oil, cinnamon, paprika, cayenne, salt, and black pepper.

Pour the spiced coconut oil over the nuts in the large bowl. Using your hands or a large spoon, toss the nuts in the spiced oil, making sure to evenly coat all of the nuts. Spread the nuts in an even layer on the lined baking sheet.

Bake the nuts, stirring and tossing occasionally, until toasted, 25 to 30 minutes.

Remove the nuts from the oven and let them cool to room temperature. Serve.

Store any leftover nuts in an airtight container in the refrigerator for up to 5 days.

Nutritional analysis per serving (4 tablespoons nuts): *Calories: 206, Fat: 19 g, Saturated Fat: 4 g, Cholesterol: 0 mg, Fiber: 3 g, Protein: 5 g, Carbohydrates: 8 g, Sodium: 66 mg*

ROASTED GARLIC WITH OLIVE OIL AND ROSEMARY

When a whole head of garlic is roasted slowly in the oven, the garlic softens and sweetens into a mild, creamy paste. It loses all its sharp pungency, and mellows out into a fragrant, gentler version of itself. Roasted garlic can be used as a spread, mixed into sauces and dressings, or added to pureed vegetables and soups.

Makes: about 75 ml
Prep Time: 5 minutes
Cook Time: 45 minutes

- 2 heads garlic, unpeeled
- 2 teaspoons extra-virgin olive oil
- 1 rosemary sprig

Preheat the oven to 200°C/Gas 6.

Using a serrated knife, slice both heads of garlic crosswise so you have top and bottom layers, even in size.

Rub each of the four cut surfaces with the olive oil, and then place the garlic and rosemary on a sheet of aluminium foil. Wrap the garlic and rosemary in the foil to seal it up tightly, then place it directly on a shelf in the oven.

Roast the garlic until it is very soft and fragrant, about 45 minutes; when you peek inside the foil, you should see that the cut edges are turning golden brown.

Allow the heads to cool enough to handle, then squeeze the roasted garlic from the cloves and use as needed.

Store any leftover roasted garlic in an airtight container in the refrigerator for up to 5 days.

Nutritional analysis per serving (1 tablespoon): *Calories: 29, Fat: 2 g, Saturated Fat: 0 g, Cholesterol: 0 mg, Fiber: 0 g, Protein: 1 g, Carbohydrates: 3 g, Sodium: 2 mg*

LEMONY CASHEW-TAHINI DIP

This thick, hummus-style dip tastes great with raw veggie dippers, such as broccoli, carrots, red peppers, or sugar snap peas. If you add even more water, you can thin the dip into a dressing, which pairs well with kale and other hearty greens.

Serves: 4
Prep Time: 10 minutes, plus soaking time

- 140 g raw cashews
- 4 tablespoons tahini
- juice of 1 lemon
- ¼ teaspoon sea salt

Put the cashews in a bowl and cover with at least 250 ml warm water. Let sit until softened, 20 to 30 minutes.

Use a slotted spoon to transfer the soaked cashews to a food processor, making sure to reserve the cashew soaking water. Add the tahini, lemon juice, and salt to the food processor and puree the mixture, adding 4 tablespoons of the reserved cashew water through the feed tube as it is processing. If necessary, add another few tablespoons of the water until the dip is the consistency of hummus. (For a thinner dressing, add up to 120 ml more of the reserved water, a few tablespoons at a time, until the desired consistency is achieved.) Serve.

Store any leftover dip or dressing in an airtight container in the refrigerator for 3 to 5 days.

Nutritional analysis per serving (4 tablespoons): *Calories: 270, Fat: 22 g, Saturated Fat: 4 g, Cholesterol: 0 mg, Fiber: 2 g, Protein: 9 g, Carbohydrates: 14 g, Sodium: 156 mg*

SAUCES AND CONDIMENTS

MIXED BERRY SALSA

Sneaking low-glycemic berries into what are normally vegetable-based recipes provides a touch of sweetness without the harm of refined sugar. Serve this salsa with fresh vegetables such as cucumber slices, cauliflower florets, and radishes.

Serves: 4
Prep Time: 15 minutes

- 200 g strawberries, chopped
- 60 g blueberries
- 60 g raspberries
- 1 medium tomato, cored and chopped
- ⅓ red onion, chopped
- 1 or 2 jalapeño chilies, seeded and finely chopped
- ½ bunch coriander, stems removed and chopped
- 2 tablespoons fresh lime juice
- ¼ teaspoon sea salt

Combine all of the ingredients in a medium bowl, stirring gently to combine. Serve. Store any leftover salsa in an airtight container in the refrigerator for up to 5 days.

Nutritional analysis per serving (120 ml): *Calories: 45, Fat: 0 g, Saturated Fat: 0 g, Cholesterol: 0 mg, Fiber: 3 g, Protein: 1 g, Carbohydrates: 11 g, Sodium: 150 mg*

MARINARA SAUCE

This basic tomato sauce can be served over steamed vegetables or blanched shirataki noodles for a quick lunch or dinner option.

Serves: 4
Prep Time: 10 minutes
Cook Time: 40 minutes

- 1½ teaspoons olive oil
- 1 medium onion, finely chopped
- 2 garlic cloves, finely chopped
- 2 (400-g) cans chopped tomatoes
- 2 bay leaves
- ¾ teaspoon dried oregano
- ½ teaspoon dried thyme
- ½ teaspoon dried basil
- ½ teaspoon sea salt
- ¼ teaspoon freshly ground black pepper
- 2 tablespoons chopped fresh basil

In a heavy saucepan, heat the oil over medium-high heat until shimmering. Add the onion and cook, stirring frequently, until softened, 8 to 10 minutes.

Add the garlic and cook, stirring, for 30 seconds. Add the tomatoes with their juices, bay leaves, dried herbs, salt, and black pepper. Stir to combine. Let the sauce come to the boil and then reduce the heat to a simmer. Partially cover the pan and cook the sauce for 30 minutes.

Remove the bay leaves and serve, garnished with the fresh basil. Store any leftover sauce in an airtight container in the refrigerator for up to 5 days.

Nutritional analysis per serving (175 ml): *Calories: 73, Fat: 2 g, Saturated Fat: 0 g, Cholesterol: 0 mg, Fiber: 2 g, Protein: 2 g, Carbohydrates: 12 g, Sodium: 313 mg*

SESAME-COCONUT CURRY SAUCE

This peanut-free version of a classic Asian sauce can be served with grilled chicken satay, steamed vegetables, or spring rolls.

Serves: 8
Prep Time: 15 minutes
Cook Time: 15 minutes

- 1 tablespoon grapeseed oil
- 1 large garlic clove, finely chopped
- 5-cm piece ginger, peeled and grated
- 2 teaspoons curry powder
- ½ teaspoon ground turmeric
- ¼ teaspoon cayenne pepper (optional)
- 1 (400-ml) can full-fat unsweetened coconut milk
- 4 tablespoons tahini
- 4 tablespoons almond butter
- 1 tablespoon gluten-free, low-sodium tamari
- ½ teaspoon toasted sesame oil
- 1 tablespoon fresh lime juice

Warm the grapeseed oil in a saucepan over low heat. Add the garlic and ginger and sauté until soft and very fragrant, about 3 minutes. Add the curry powder, turmeric, and cayenne (if using) and sauté for another minute to toast the spices.

Add the coconut milk and whisk the sauce well to combine. Raise the heat to medium and simmer until the coconut milk has reduced in volume by one-third, about 10 minutes. Remove the pan from the heat and allow the sauce to cool for 5 minutes, then whisk in the tahini, almond butter, tamari, and sesame oil. Add the lime juice just before serving.

Store any leftover sauce in an airtight container in the fridge for 5 days.

Nutritional analysis per serving (4 tablespoons): *Calories: 210, Fat: 21 g, Saturated Fat: 10 g, Cholesterol: 0 mg, Fiber: 1 g, Protein: 4 g, Carbohydrates: 5 g, Sodium: 115 mg*

GREMOLATA WITH ALMONDS

Serve this refreshing condiment over roasted carrots or roasted asparagus; it also works beautifully as a side dish to any main course.

Serves: 6
Prep Time: 5 minutes, plus soaking time

- 140 g raw almonds
- 1 or 2 garlic cloves, halved
- 2 bunches parsley, stems removed
- grated zest of 2 lemons
- 1 teaspoon fresh lemon juice
- ¼ teaspoon sea salt
- pinch of freshly ground black pepper

Soak the almonds in a small bowl of warm water until softened, about 30 minutes.

Drain the almonds and transfer to a food processor. Process until finely ground, about 1 minute. Add the garlic, parsley, lemon zest, lemon juice, salt, and black pepper and process until the mixture is crumbly and finely chopped, 30 seconds to 1 minute. Serve.

Store any leftover gremolata in an airtight container in the refrigerator for up to 5 days.

Nutritional analysis per serving (4 tablespoons): *Calories: 150, Fat: 12 g, Saturated Fat: 1 g, Cholesterol: 0 mg, Fiber: 4 g, Protein: 6 g, Carbohydrates: 7 g, Sodium: 110 mg*

KALE PESTO

Baby kale makes for a fun alternative to traditional basil pesto. The lemon zest and juice bring a fresh, bright flavor to the pesto while keeping it dairy-free.

Serves: 6
Prep Time: 10 minutes

- 1 garlic clove, halved
- 2 tablespoons pine nuts
- grated zest and juice of 1 large lemon
- 150 g baby kale
- 4 tablespoons extra-virgin olive oil
- ¼ teaspoon sea salt
- ¼ teaspoon freshly ground black pepper

In a food processor, pulse the garlic and pine nuts until finely chopped. Add the lemon zest and juice. Add the kale and pulse until coarsely chopped. With the machine running, add the oil through the feed tube and puree until almost smooth. Season with the salt and black pepper and puree again.

Store any leftover pesto in an airtight container in the refrigerator for up to 5 days.

Nutritional analysis per serving (4 tablespoons): *Calories: 110, Fat: 11 g, Saturated Fat: 1.5 g, Cholesterol: 0 mg, Fiber: 1 g, Protein: 1 g, Carbohydrates: 2 g, Sodium: 100 mg*

CHIMICHURRI

This green sauce originated in Argentina and is traditionally served on meat. This version, packed with citrus and fresh herb flavors, works well on fish and chicken, too.

Serves: 6
Prep Time: 10 minutes

- 2 bunches parsley, stems removed
- 1 bunch coriander, stems included
- ½ bunch mint, stems removed
- 2 oil-packed anchovies
- 1 tablespoon capers, rinsed
- 1 garlic clove, halved
- 2 tablespoons extra-virgin olive oil
- grated zest and juice of ½ lemon
- ¼ teaspoon sea salt
- pinch of freshly ground black pepper

Combine all of the ingredients in a food processor and blend until smooth. Store any leftover sauce in an airtight container in the refrigerator for up to 5 days.

Nutritional analysis per serving (2 tablespoons): *Calories: 50, Fat: 5 g, Saturated Fat: 0.5 g, Cholesterol: 0 mg, Fiber: 1 g, Protein: 1 g, Carbohydrates: 2 g, Sodium: 200 mg*

CASHEW "RICOTTA CHEESE"

Cashews contain magnesium, copper, manganese, zinc, healthy essential fatty acids, and protein, and they tend to be hypoallergenic so most people can tolerate them easily. Serve this spread with fresh vegetables such as peppers, celery, or sugar snap peas as a healthy alternative to dairy cheese.

Makes: about 500 ml
Prep Time: 5 minutes, plus soaking time

- 275 g raw cashews
- 2 tablespoons extra-virgin olive oil
- 4 teaspoons fresh lemon juice
- 1 teaspoon sea salt

Soak the cashews in a bowl of hot water for at least 1 hour at room temperature or up to 24 hours in the refrigerator. Drain the cashews and place them in a food processor, along with the olive oil, lemon juice, salt, and 4 tablespoons of warm water. Process the ingredients until a smooth paste forms; you may need to add a bit more water, depending on how long you soaked the cashews. Serve.

Store any leftover "cheese" in an airtight container in the refrigerator for up to 3 days.

Nutritional analysis per serving (4 tablespoons): *Calories: 210, Fat: 18 g, Saturated Fat: 3 g, Cholesterol: 0 mg, Fiber: 1 g, Protein: 6 g, Carbohydrates: 11 g, Sodium: 290 mg*

Spicy Tomatillo-Avocado Sauce

This sauce, when chilled, is a wonderful substitute for sour cream in Tex-Mex dishes, and it adds a bit of richness as a garnish for a pureed vegetable soup. It also takes well to the addition of spices, so feel free to change it up a bit. I like to add cumin, chili powder, or curry powder. Try experimenting with your favorite spices.

Serves: 6
Prep Time: 10 minutes
Cook Time: 15 minutes

- 4 small tomatillos, husks removed
- 1 jalapeño chili, seeded and halved
- 1 avocado, peeled and stoned
- juice of 1 lime
- ¼ teaspoon sea salt

Fill a 3-liter saucepan with water and add the tomatillos and jalapeño. Bring the water to the boil over medium-high heat, then reduce to a simmer and cook until the tomatillos are tender, 7 to 10 minutes. With a slotted spoon, transfer the tomatillos and jalapeño to a blender, and puree until smooth. Add the avocado, lime juice, and salt and continue to puree until a thick sauce forms. Serve.

Store any leftover sauce in an airtight container, with greaseproof paper pressed against the surface of the sauce to prevent discoloration, for up to 3 days.

Nutritional analysis per serving (4 tablespoons): *Calories: 60, Fat: 5 g, Saturated Fat: 0.5 g, Cholesterol: 0 mg, Fiber: 3 g, Protein: 1 g, Carbohydrates: 5 g, Sodium: 105 mg*

Salsa Roja

Serve this salsa as a dip with cucumber slices and other mild vegetables. It is also great swirled into soup, used as a salad dressing, or spooned over meat.

Serves: 4
Prep Time: 10 minutes, plus soaking time

- 6 dried chilies
- 3 tomatoes, roughly chopped
- ¼ red onion, chopped
- 1 garlic clove, halved
- 1½ tablespoons cider vinegar
- ¼ teaspoon sea salt

Put the dried chilies in a bowl and add enough boiling water to cover. Soak them until softened, 20 to 30 minutes.

Remove the chilies from the bowl with a slotted spoon, reserving 4 tablespoons of the soaking water.

Peel open the chilies and remove the stems and seeds. Put the chilies in a food processor, along with the tomatoes, onion, garlic, vinegar, and salt. Process the mixture, adding the reserved chili soaking water through the feed tube. Blend until the salsa is smooth, 1 to 2 minutes. Serve.

Store any leftover salsa in an airtight container in the refrigerator for up to 5 days.

Nutritional analysis per serving (120 ml): *Calories: 35, Fat: 0 g, Saturated Fat: 0 g, Cholesterol: 0 mg, Fiber: 1 g, Protein: 1 g, Carbohydrates: 7 g, Sodium: 160 mg*

ROASTED PEPPER AND RED ONION RELISH

Impress your guests the next time you have company over with this savory, slightly sweet relish. Spread it on top of fresh vegetables or use it to dress up a plain roast chicken or steamed fish. If you don't have a slow cooker, you can bake the roasted vegetables in a covered cast-iron casserole at 150°C/Gas 2 for 3½ hours.

Makes: about 500 ml
Prep Time: 20 minutes
Cook Time: 12 hours (unattended), plus 30 minutes

- 6 red peppers, seeded and cut into 1-cm-thick strips
- 2 jalapeño chilies, seeded and thinly sliced (optional)
- 5 red onions, cut crosswise into 1-cm-thick slices and separated into rings
- 4 tablespoons extra-virgin olive oil
- sea salt

Preheat the oven to 260°C/Gas highest setting.

Line two rimmed baking sheets with aluminium foil. Place half of the peppers and onions on the baking sheets and toss the vegetables on each sheet with 1 tablespoon of the olive oil and a pinch of salt. Roast the peppers and onions until they are tender and browning at the edges, 15 to 17 minutes, rotating the sheets halfway through cooking. Transfer the vegetables to a 6-liter slow cooker.

Roast the second batch of peppers and onions in the same way, again tossing each sheet with 1 tablespoon of the olive oil and a pinch of salt. Transfer to the slow cooker.

Once all of the vegetables have been added, cook on low for 12 hours. Serve.

Store any leftover relish in an airtight container in the refrigerator for up to 2 weeks.

Nutritional analysis per serving (4 tablespoons): *Calories: 150, Fat: 10 g, Saturated Fat: 1.5 g, Cholesterol: 0 mg, Fiber: 4 g, Protein: 2 g, Carbohydrates: 16 g, Sodium: 200 mg*

MAYONNAISE

Homemade mayo tastes so much better than the kind from a jar, and if you make it in the blender, it's super fast! Since raw eggs are used, be sure to buy organic eggs for this recipe.

Makes: about 250 ml
Prep Time: 5 minutes

- 1 large omega-3 egg
- 4 teaspoons fresh lemon juice
- 1 teaspoon Dijon mustard
- ¼ teaspoon sea salt
- ¼ teaspoon freshly ground black pepper
- 250 ml extra-virgin olive oil

In a blender or food processor, combine the egg, lemon juice, mustard, salt, and black pepper and blend until well combined, 1 to 2 minutes.

With the blender still running, slowly add the oil in a steady stream through the hole in the lid and continue to blend until the mayo is thick and smooth. Serve.

Store any leftover mayonnaise in an airtight container in the refrigerator for up to 1 week.

Nutritional analysis per serving (1 tablespoon): *Calories: 125, Fat: 14 g, Saturated Fat: 2 g, Cholesterol: 14 mg, Fiber: 0 g, Protein: 1 g, Carbohydrates: 0 g, Sodium: 45 mg*

SPICES, RUBS, AND STOCKS

RAS EL HANOUT

Ras el hanout is a Middle Eastern spice mix available at some supermarkets, but it's easy enough to make your own. Use this in the Pomegranate Chicken recipe (page 188); it also makes a tasty rub for all kinds of meat, poultry, and fish.

Makes: about 3 tablespoons
Prep Time: 5 minutes

- 2 teaspoons ground cumin
- 1 teaspoon ground ginger
- 1 teaspoon ground cinnamon
- 1 teaspoon ground coriander
- 1 teaspoon sea salt
- ¾ teaspoon freshly ground black pepper
- ½ teaspoon cayenne pepper
- ½ teaspoon ground allspice

Combine all of the ingredients in a small bowl and mix well. Store in an airtight container in a cool, dark place for up to 1 month.

Nutritional analysis per serving (1 teaspoon): *Calories: 5, Fat: 0 g, Saturated Fat: 0 g, Cholesterol: 0 mg, Fiber: 1 g, Protein: 0 g, Carbohydrates: 1 g, Sodium: 290 mg*

DR. HYMAN'S GO-TO SPICE RUB

Keep a batch of this spice rub easily accessible in your pantry to elevate any weeknight meal featuring fish, poultry, or meat to an extraordinary dining experience.

Makes: about 4 tablespoons
Prep Time: 5 minutes

- 2 teaspoons ground turmeric
- 2 teaspoons smoked or sweet paprika
- 2 teaspoons ground coriander
- 2 teaspoons ground cumin
- 2 teaspoons ground ginger
- ½ teaspoon ground cloves
- 2 teaspoons sea salt

Combine all of the ingredients in a small bowl and mix well. Store in an airtight container in a cool, dark place for up to 1 month.

Nutritional analysis per serving (1 teaspoon): *Calories: 5, fat: 0 g, Saturated Fat: 0 g, Cholesterol: 0 mg, Fiber: 0 g, Protein: 0 g, Carbohydrates: 1 g, Sodium: 382 mg*

THAI GREEN CURRY PASTE

Full of spice and flavor, this paste is perfect in my Thai Green Curry with Soft-Shell Crabs (page 143).

Makes: about 175 ml
Prep Time: 20 minutes
Cook Time: 3 minutes

- 1 tablespoon coriander seeds
- 1 tablespoon cumin seeds
- ½ teaspoon black peppercorns
- 4 to 6 green bird's eye or serrano chilies, seeded
- 1 lemongrass stalk, roughly chopped
- 3 large shallots, roughly chopped
- 15 garlic cloves, halved
- 3 (5-cm) pieces ginger, peeled and roughly chopped
- 1 bunch parsley, stems removed
- 2 tablespoons fish sauce
- 1 teaspoon sea salt

Toast the coriander seeds, cumin seeds, and peppercorns in a large frying pan over medium heat until fragrant and beginning to brown, 2 to 3 minutes, stirring constantly. Transfer to a plate to cool.

In a spice grinder, grind the cooled spices until a powder forms. Set aside.

In the bowl of a food processor, combine the chilies, lemongrass, shallots, garlic, ginger, parsley, fish sauce, and salt. Process, scraping down the sides of the bowl, until the mixture is a smooth paste, about 2 minutes. If the food processor begins to warm up (feel the side of the machine), give it a 5-minute break to cool down; do not overwork the engine. Once the mixture is smooth, add the ground spices and continue to process until combined.

Store the paste in an airtight container in the refrigerator for up to 7 days.

Nutritional analysis per serving (1 tablespoon): *Calories: 35, Fat: 0 g, Saturated Fat: 0 g, Cholesterol: 0 mg, Fiber: 1 g, Protein: 2 g, Carbohydrates: 7 g, Sodium: 582 mg*

Herb Salt

Herb salt is a great way to customize your favorite dishes. You can use a variety of fresh herbs (experiment by mixing and matching) to make different blends that will add kick to vegetables, meat, and fish. The salt is quick to assemble and lasts a long time.

Makes: about 500 g
Prep Time: 10 minutes
Cook Time: 2½ hours

- 500 g sea salt
- 3 tablespoons chopped fresh thyme
- 1 tablespoon chopped fresh rosemary
- 1 tablespoon chopped fresh tarragon

Preheat the oven to 100°C/Gas lowest setting.

Combine all of the ingredients in a bowl. Evenly spread the salt mixture on a rimmed baking sheet. Bake, stirring occasionally, until the herbs are no longer moist, about 2½ hours.

Allow the salt to cool completely, then transfer to an airtight container. Store in a cool, dark place for up 1 month.

Nutritional analysis per serving (¼ teaspoon): *Calories: 0, Fat: 0 g, Saturated Fat: 0 g, Cholesterol: 0 mg, Fiber: 0 g, Protein: 0 g, Carbohydrates: 0 g, Sodium: 480 mg.*

VEGETABLE-HERB STOCK

Making homemade stock is a simple, fun way to enjoy nutrient-dense ingredients. Make a double batch and store half in the freezer—once you taste it, you won't miss the store-bought version for a second.

Serves: 4
Prep Time: 15 minutes
Cook Time: 1 hour and 15 minutes

- 2 fennel bulbs with fronds, sliced
- 2 carrots, roughly chopped
- 2 onions, roughly chopped
- 300 g chestnut mushrooms, trimmed and halved
- 50 g spinach or other greens
- 5 garlic cloves, halved
- 1 bunch parsley, stems included
- 1 large rosemary sprig
- 5 to 6 thyme sprigs
- 2 bay leaves
- 1 teaspoon sea salt
- 1 teaspoon black peppercorns
- 1 teaspoon coconut aminos or gluten-free, low-sodium tamari

Combine all of the ingredients in a large saucepan. Add 2.5 to 3 liters of water to the pan, enough to cover the vegetables. Don't worry about some veggies poking out; they will sink down during the cooking.

Bring the water to the boil over high heat; reduce the heat to a simmer and cook for 60 to 75 minutes.

Let the stock cool a bit, then strain out the solids by pouring the stock through a colander placed over a large bowl. Discard the solids.

Pour the vegetable stock into airtight containers and store in the refrigerator for up to 3 days or in the freezer for up to 6 months.

Nutritional analysis per serving (250 ml): *Calories: 5, Fat: 0 g, Saturated Fat: 0 g, Cholesterol: 0 mg, Fiber: 0 g, Protein: 0 g, Carbohydrates: 2 g, Sodium: 200 mg*

8

Healthy Meal Plans

Now that you have the tools and tips and have been introduced to all these new ingredients, you might be wondering which meals work best together to create complete meals. I hope the following suggestions help you create delicious meal plans for your family and friends. *Bon appétit!*

LUNCH AND DINNER IDEAS

Creamy Herbed Tahini Dip, Rocket and Fennel Salad, and Ginger-Lemon Chicken with Spinach

Heirloom Tomato, Cucumber, and Radish Salad, steamed carrots with Gremolata with Almonds, and Lebanese-Style Lamb Stew

Onion-Leek Soup, Niçoise Salad with Poached Salmon, and Pepper Mini Quiches

Chicken Spring Rolls with Almond Sauce, Spicy Garlic Aubergine with Mint, and Thai Green Curry with Soft-Shell Crabs

Taco Salad with Skirt Steak, Spicy Cauliflower Sauté, and Spicy Mocktail

Thai Tofu and Avocado Salad with Chili-Lime Dressing, Fried "Rice" with Prawns, and Asian-Spiced Salmon Cakes

Deviled Eggs, Moroccan Chicken and Vegetable Stew, and Steamed Vegetables with Lemon Aioli

Roasted Vegetables with Artichoke Hummus, Courgette Ribbons with Pearl Onions and Cardamom, Miso-Marinated Cod with Fresh Basil and Pak Choi, and Cauliflower "Rice"

Warm Herbed Olives, Stuffed Tomatoes, and Chili-Spiced Turkey Meatloaf with Roasted Carrot Salad

BRUNCH IDEAS

Blueberry-Nut Smoothie, Cherry Tomato and Tofu Salad, and Vegetable Hash with Fried Eggs

Açai Smoothie, Crustless Asparagus Quiche, and Turkey Sausage Patties

Jicama Fries, Chicken Salad in Chicory Cups, Spinach-Mushroom-Asparagus Strata, and Creamy Berry Smoothie

Heirloom Tomato, Cucumber, and Radish Salad, Garlic and Chili Tenderstem Broccoli with Soft-Boiled Eggs, and Almond-Berry Smoothie

Egg Salad in Chicory Spears, Grilled Chicken with Basil Pesto, and Strawberry-Almond-Coconut Smoothie

AFTER THE 10-DAY DETOX DIET

Congratulations! You have given yourself a gift—the gift of real food and optimal health. The main idea behind *The 10-Day Detox Diet* and *The 10-Day Detox Diet Cookbook* is to help you connect the dots between what you eat and how you feel, and to provide a way for you to experience the power of food as medicine. But now what? Now you can reintroduce foods (but only real foods) to your diet and monitor how you feel. I hope you never go back to eating processed, industrial science projects masquerading as food, or to pharmacological doses of sugar and flour. My hope is that you stick with real, whole, fresh food. My hope is for you to introduce beans, grains, and even small amounts of dairy and gluten and sugar (as a treat) and see how you feel. You now have a fresh start, an opportunity to transition to a new way of eating and to notice how your body likes (or doesn't) certain foods, like gluten and dairy.

Depending on your goals, there are different options for transitioning off *The 10-Day Detox Diet*. I have created a free downloadable guide—*The 10-Day Detox Diet Cookbook Companion Guide*—with detailed guidelines on how to transition safely while enjoying a wide variety of delicious foods. The guide includes instructions on how to discover which transition plan is best for you, how to safely reintroduce foods without getting sick, and how to track their effects on your health. And I have also included a few delicious, easy recipes for the Transition Phase. Please go to www.10daydetox.com/tools to download your free guide!

This book is meant to help you figure out how to change your life through food. Whether you are just beginning to experiment with simple ways to prepare basic foods or expanding your repertoire to include new tastes and ingredients, I hope this book provides the road map, the tools and the inspiration. I had two main goals in writing this book.

First, I want to encourage you to cook real, delicious, and inspiring meals—for yourself, your family, or your entire community. As you stick to real foods prepared simply, you'll notice the pounds come off, the cravings disappear, and just about every aspect of your health improve.

And second, I want you to feel so great after the 10 days that you'll never want to return to the food desert from which you came. You will want to stay nourished and healthy. You'll want to continue healing yourself, your family, and your community through food. And not just for 10 days, but for the rest of your life.

After all, better health doesn't start and end in 10 days. It's a life-long journey. I've set out to make that journey both doable and delicious. Bon voyage, and *bon appétit!*

Acknowledgments

This cookbook is the work of many passionate souls who love food and are committed to transforming how we grow, produce, and consume food.

The vision started with one mission: to create simple, delicious, healing meals that help people experience the power of food. The power of food to delight the palate, invigorate the senses, and reboot the body. The power of real, whole, fresh food to help people see the connection between what they eat and how they feel, and realize that they are only ten days away from health and happiness.

But to do that, I needed to create inspired and delectable recipes that are easy and fun to make. So I gathered an amazing team. The team was led by Anne McLaughlin, who ensured that everything made sense and kept me on track. Lizzy Swick provided the oversight to make sure that my vision of healing, detoxifying ingredients was incorporated into each and every recipe. Lauren Zander and Amy Teuteberg created the Dinner Conversations, a way to bring love and connection and laughter into every meal.

Most important, the team at Luvo designed and created the healing recipes. Thank you, team Luvo: Christine Day, Chief Executive Officer; Stephen Sidwell, Founder; John Mitchell, Chief Innovation Officer and Executive Chef; Samantha Cassetty, Director of Nutrition; Margaret Wetzler, Director of Culinary Marketing; Eunice Choi, Project Manager, Culinary Marketing; Diane Maynard, Art Director; Diane Elander, Food

Stylist; Bruce James, Photographer; Andrea Lynn, Emma Feigenbaum, Erica Wides, and Genevieve Ko, Recipe Developers; and Brooks Halliday and Faryl Amadeus, Recipe Testers.

Of course, I could not have created all this without the love and support of my team at Little, Brown, especially my editor, Tracy Behar. Thank you for believing in the future of food and health and helping me make it a reality. My success is in large part because of my long-time believer, supporter, advocate, and agent, Richard Pine. Thank you for being part of the change.

Finally, thank *you* for taking back your kitchens, for taking a step closer to a vibrant, healthy life through the power of food. Cooking is the ultimate revolutionary act—food that we make ourselves can be simple, quick, inexpensive, and delicious. And cooking real food can transform everything that is ailing us as a society, because it changes how we produce and consume food—taking it out of the hands of Big Food and Big Ag and putting it back in your hands, where it belongs.

Resources

FURTHER READING AND RESOURCES FROM MARK HYMAN, MD

Mark Hyman's Websites

www.drhyman.com
www.10daydetox.com
www.bloodsugarsolution.com

The UltraWellness Center

55 Pittsfield Road, Suite 9
Lenox Commons
Lenox, MA 01240
(413) 637-9991
www.ultrawellnesscenter.com

I founded and am the medical director of this center. Our team of experienced functional medicine physicians, nutritionists, nurses, and health coaches guide you through diet and lifestyle modifications, as well as specialized testing, nutritional supplementation, and medications.

Cleveland Clinic Center for Functional Medicine

9500 Euclid Avenue / H-18
Cleveland, OH 44195
(216) 445-6900 or toll-free at (844) 833-0126

I am the director of this center. Our team of experienced functional medicine physicians, nutritionists, nurses, and health coaches guide you through diet and lifestyle modifications, as well as specialized testing, nutritional supplementation, and medications.

Books and Programs

The Blood Sugar Solution 10-Day Detox Diet (Book and Public Television Special)

www.10daydetox.com

The Blood Sugar Solution (Book and Public Television Special)

www.bloodsugarsolution.com

The UltraMind Solution (Book and Public Television Special)

Six Weeks to an UltraMind (Audio/DVD Program)

The Daniel Plan

www.danielplan.com

The Daniel Plan Cookbook

UltraCalm (Audio Program)

UltraMetabolism (Book and Public Television Special)

The UltraMetabolism Cookbook (Book)

The UltraSimple Diet (Book)

The UltraSimple Challenge (DVD Coaching Program)

The UltraThyroid Solution (Ebook)

UltraPrevention (Book)

Five Forces of Wellness (Audio Program)

The Detox Box (Audio/DVD Detoxification Program)

Nutrigenomics

THE 10-DAY DETOX DIET TOOLS AND RESOURCES PAGE

For additional information on resources listed in this book, please see below or visit www.10daydetox.com/tools for additional online resources, including:

Health and Testing Resources

- Basic lab tests (lists which lab tests you need to check for diabesity)
- Online versions of *The Blood Sugar Solution* Diabesity Quiz, Toxicity Quiz, and Food Addiction Quiz

- The *How to Work with Your Doctor to Get What You Need* downloadable guide
- Testing tools (including BMI calculator, glucose monitors, FitBit Wi-Fi Smart Scale, blood pressure monitors, and personal movement trackers)
- The 10-Day Detox Online Health Tracker and Online Journal
- The 10-Day Detox Supplements
- The 10-Day Detox Diet Coaching App
- The 10-Day Detox Diet Tool Kit for Success

10-Day Detox Community Resources

- The 10-Day Detox Challenge
- The 10-Day Detox Community
- How to find a local food co-op
- Life coaching resources

Lifestyle Resources

- Exercise and yoga resources
- The *UltraCalm* guided relaxation program
- Meditation and breathing resources
- Herbal resources
- Stress Management Guide

Food and Nutrition Guides, Support, and Meals

- Access to nutrition coaching support
- Downloadable 10-Day Detox Diet Shopping List
- Brand recommendations for Emergency Life Pack
- The *Restaurant Rescue Guide*
- The 10-Day Detox Diet Vegetarian and Vegan Guide
- Luvo's 10-Day Detox Meals (delicious frozen home meals): luvoinc.com/10-day-detox

General Index

Recipe Index

About the Author

MARK HYMAN, MD, has dedicated his career to identifying and addressing the root causes of chronic illness through a groundbreaking whole-systems medicine approach known as Functional Medicine. He is a family physician, an eight-time #1 *New York Times* bestselling author, and an internationally recognized leader in his field. Through his private practice, education efforts, writing, research, advocacy, and public-policy work, he strives to improve access to Functional Medicine and to widen the understanding and practice of it, empowering others to stop managing symptoms and instead treat the underlying causes of illness, thereby also tackling our chronic-disease epidemic.

Dr. Hyman is Chairman of the Institute for Functional Medicine, and was awarded its 2009 Linus Pauling Award for Leadership in Functional Medicine. He is also director of the Cleveland Clinic Center for Functional Medicine. He is on the Board of Directors of the Center for Mind-Body Medicine and a faculty member of its Food As Medicine training program, as well as a member of the Board of Advisors of Mehmet Oz's HealthCorps, which tackles the obesity epidemic by educating the student body in American high schools about nutrition, fitness, and mental resilience. He is a volunteer for Partners in Health, with whom he worked immediately after the earthquake in Haiti and continues to help rebuild the country's health care system there. He was featured on *60 Minutes* for his work there.

Dr. Hyman has testified before the White House Commission on Complementary and Alternative Medicine and has consulted with the

Surgeon General on diabetes prevention. He has testified before the Senate Working Group on Health Care Reform on functional medicine and participated in the White House Forum on Prevention and Wellness in June 2009. Dr. Hyman was nominated by Senator Tom Harkin for the President's Advisory Group on Prevention, Health Promotion, and Integrative and Public Health, a twenty-five-person group to advise the administration and the new National Council on Prevention, Health Promotion, and Public Health. With Drs. Dean Ornish and Michael Roizen, Dr. Hyman crafted and helped to introduce the Take Back Your Health Act of 2009 into the United States Senate, to provide for reimbursement of lifestyle treatment of chronic disease. He is an international speaker and presented at TEDMED, the World Economic Forum and the Clinton Foundation's Health Matters Conference, as well as the Clinton Global Initiative America. He continues to work in Washington on health reform, recently testifying before a congressional hearing on functional medicine, nutrition, and the use of dietary supplements.

Through his work with corporations, church groups, and government entities, such as CIGNA, the Veterans Administration, Google, and Saddleback Church, he is helping to improve health outcomes and reduce medical costs around the world. He initiated and is a key participant in the ongoing development of a faith-based initiative that enrolled over 15,000 people at Saddleback Church in a healthy lifestyle program and research study where the congregation lost 250,000 pounds in the first year. In recognition of his efforts, he was recently awarded the Council on Litigation Management's 2010 Professionalism Award, citing individuals who have demonstrated leadership by example in the highest standard of their profession. He also received the American College of Nutrition 2009 Communication and Media Award for his contribution to promoting better understanding of nutrition science. He has been featured on *The Dr. Oz Show, CBS This Morning, 60 Minutes,* CNN, and MSNBC. He was inducted into the Books for a Better Life Hall of Fame in 2015.

Dr. Hyman is founder and medical director of the UltraWellness Center in Lenox, Massachusetts, where he directs a team of physicians, nutritionists, and nurses who utilize a comprehensive approach to health.

Before starting his practice, he was co–medical director at Canyon Ranch Lenox, one of the world's leading health resorts. While at Canyon Ranch, he coauthored the *New York Times* bestseller *UltraPrevention: The 6-Week Plan That Will Make You Healthy for Life* (Scribner) — winner of the Books for a Better Life Award honoring the best self-improvement books each year. He has since written *UltraMetabolism: The Simple Plan for Automatic Weight Loss, The UltraMetabolism Cookbook, The UltraMind Solution, The UltraSimple Diet, The Blood Sugar Solution, The Blood Sugar Solution Cookbook, The Blood Sugar Solution 10-Day Detox Diet*, and *Eat Fat Get Thin,* as well as co-authored *The Daniel Plan* and *The Daniel Plan Cookbook,* all #1 *New York Times* bestsellers. Dr. Hyman graduated with a B.A. from Cornell University and magna cum laude from the Ottawa University School of Medicine. He completed his residency at the University of San Francisco's program in Family Medicine at the Community Hospital of Santa Rosa. Please join him in helping us all take back our health at www .drhyman.com, follow him on twitter @markhymanmd, and see him on Facebook at facebook.com/drmarkhyman.